NATURAL MEDICINE

For a Healthy Mind and Body
And a Healthy World

Bonnie Camo MD

2

NATURAL MEDICINE

For a Healthy Mind and Body, and a Healthy World

Bonnie Camo MD

To all my patients, who taught me as much as I taught them.

Acknowledgements

I would like to thank Sidney M Baker MD, Phillip Bonnet MD, Luc de Schepper MD, Sharon Downey, Les Fehmi PhD, Joan Goldstein PhD, Lynne Hewitt RN, Maureen McDonnell RN, Dorothy Mullen, and James Neubrander MD, for reading all or part of the manuscript and offering insightful suggestions that greatly improved the clarity and accuracy of the presentation. I would also like to thank my editor Barbara Bergstrom for her tireless work and advice that enabled this book to come to fruition.

Table of Contents   page

6

Forward
By Phillip Bonnet MD

"The physician's high and only mission is to restore the sick to health, to cure, as it is termed."
Samuel Hahnemann, <u>Organon of Medicine</u>, aphorism # 1.

Amazingly, in <u>Natural Medicine,</u> Bonnie Camo MD raised the bar by providing a tool whereby people can, with lifestyle changes, nutrition, and homeopathy, become their own physicians, and not only restore themselves to health, but prevent illness in the first place.

Dr. Camo alerts us to a greater threat to our existence than President Eisenhower's warning of the military-industrial complex's threat to America's democracy. Corporate interests, she writes, in their soulless pursuit of profit, are destroying not only our health but also life on this planet as we know it. <u>We are teetering on the brink of disaster</u>. <u>Natural Medicine</u> (a treasure trove of pearls of wisdom, physical, psychological, as well as spiritual), with its alert to the danger and the beginnings of a solution, arrives well past the 11th hour.

Dr. Camo and I both went to Hahnemann Medical School, interned at Allentown General Hospital, had the privilege of being mentored by Dr. Carl Pfeiffer, and were led by our patients to the practice of homeopathy. We became more acquainted when I drove her to a talk by Dr. Luc DeSchepper (who was to become her homeopathic mentor), but I did not realize what kindred spirits we were until I read her book.

Starting with the introduction, she engages us with her success in overcoming her training as an allopathic (mainstream) physician, and utilizing homeopathic as well as other holistic interventions, by listening to her patients.

The pharmaceutical industry's success in brainwashing, first the medical establishment, and now the general public, into believing that it is sensible to think that the question is "which is the best <u>drug</u> to suppress this symptom," rather than " what is this symptom telling us about the underlying problem," is referenced throughout. With their lobbyists in Washington gaining control of the FDA, being allowed to label promotion as education, big Pharma together with the insurance industry has created a situation in which exponentially increasing resources are being squandered on "healthcare." All the while we are experiencing progressive deterioration of our wellness. Richly documented throughout the text, our becoming increasingly toxic from pollutants and food additives, as well as a multiplicity of medication, is most explicitly detailed in the Afterword. For example, it is now commonplace to find persons so confused and befuddled that they are diagnosed as suffering from Alzheimer's disease, and have the situation resolve by getting the poor soul to stop taking some of their drugs.

 Early in the book she provides documentation of many dangers from processed food and corporate farming, with topics as diverse as the obesigenic effect of pesticides, to the inflammatory dangers of excess omega-6 fat. The healthy balance of equal amounts of omega-3 and 6 has deteriorated in some American diets to twenty times more omega-6! Dr. Camo's work is not merely a diatribe against food additives and processed food. She also offers helpful solutions.   The notion that healthy eating is "boring crunchy granola" is brilliantly dispelled in the mouthwatering chapter 8, "The Real Mediterranean Diet." In Chapter 7, Dr. Camo lays a foundation for a new world order, one in which the old misogynistic male-dominated hierarchical order is supplanted by an egalitarian cooperative matriarchal one. Her truths are not always comforting; I was disquieted by the fact that fifty percent of women prefer chocolate to sex!

While most medical practitioners would have to confess that nasal decongestants are more addictive than cocaine or heroin (one use provides immediate symptomatic relief as well as irritation to the mucosal membrane necessitating further use,) I never stopped to reflect on the fact that the PDR (Physician's Desk Reference, the text provided by drug companies to give medical doctors the necessary information to properly prescribe medications) fails to offer information as to how to discontinue drugs, until it was pointed out by Dr. Camo. How many medical doctors have any inkling that NSAIDS (non-steroidal anti-inflammatories, the medications most commonly used to treat arthritic disorders) interfere with rebuilding cartilage, thereby reducing pain while worsening the problem? Or similarly that antidepressants over time cause reduction of the very receptors they stimulate, "using pharmaceuticals to treat unpleasant life events can turn sadness into legal drug addiction"

Homeopathy is a system of medical therapeutics first discovered by Dr. Samuel Hahnemann in the late 1700's, coming into use hundreds of years before we understood the scientific principles (quantum mechanics) necessary to comprehend how it works. In the beginning of Part Three, Dr. Camo offers an exquisite explanation, comprehensible to any intelligent reader, as to how homeopathy works.

It would be reasonable to think that Hahnemann Medical School, (founded by Constantine Herring, "The Father of American Homeopathy," and named in honor of his mentor,) would have provided a foundation in homeopathy; however, the only credit given was "Homeopathy has gone the way of the horse and buggy. Its epitaph 'they killed far fewer in their day'." Having learned that the effectiveness of homeopathy is based on a placebo response, I teased my father (a radiologist) by saying, " Did you know that back when you were practicing homeopathy you were practicing placebo medicine?" He responded, "I don't know about that but, it did work and never had the side effects of what's being used today. We threw the baby out with the bathwater when we left homeopathy behind." I was still young enough to think I knew everything and dismissed what he said, thinking that if homeopathy was half as good as he insisted, he would still be in general practice. When I became interested in cerebral allergies and neutralization therapy, my father said he was very pleased that I was

10

now practicing a form of homeopathy: diluting the substance that caused the problem to the point where it would help solve the problem. It was not until many years later, when a patient with whom I tried my best and failed came to tell me that it was homeopathy that made a difference, that I decided to reconsider homeopathy and start to seriously study it.

Natural Medicine is organized both to be a good introduction for any intelligent layperson and enriching reading even for a practicing homeopath. Here, as throughout, Dr. Camo provides an excellent bibliography for any student to go much deeper.

In medical school I was taught that we were being trained to treat illness and that the word "heal" was to be avoided, because it was suspiciously nonscientific. Over time I came to realize that treating mostly involved suppression of symptoms (my dentist once teased me, "You MDs consider health to be an acceptable level of misery"), while healing should be a physician's real goal.

When we think of disease as a manifestation of the physical and energetic aspects of ourselves being in disharmony, the question is not whether our body is the temple in which our spirit dwells, or the physical materialization of our energetic body, but "What change is necessary for us to evolve toward our greater potential?" The symptom is not the problem, but is the body's solution to a deeper problem. As a physician I feel most encouraged when a patient informs me that their illness was "hell to go through, but dealing with it has enriched me to the point that I now realize it was really a blessing in disguise."

There is considerable scientific debate as to whether we are using only 2% or 10% of our potential brainpower, but there is general agreement that even the most the most actualized of us is operating way below our potential. Part Five of Natural Medicine offers several tools for assisting us in closing that disparity.   Breath, light, yoga, and meditation are among the useful modalities presented; we are even given a scientific basis for the truth that being helpful to others is the best source of real happiness.

Just as we may take a meaning from a painting or a poem different than intended by the artist or poet, so a patient may understand their recovery in a different light than the physician. At the end of several chapters patients' stories are presented. The theoretical is put into concrete focus by having several people give their accounts of utilizing natural interventions to overcome chronic illness. By having them describe both the suffering and recovery in their own words, Dr. Camo helps us understand how healing works. Sufficiently detailed to give a realistic clinical picture, while concise enough to hold one's interest, these stories provide examples of the integrated use of the various modalities presented in the chapters. While the AMA was initially formed for the explicit purpose of eradicating homeopathy, the real destruction of homeopathy (in America) came from homeopaths fighting with each other. As patients heal they become healers themselves, and here they are allowed to present homeopathy as they have come to understand it.

In The Biotypes of Alcoholism, Dr. Camo shares her research in the utilization of nutritional intervention in alleviating this affliction. I found her comments on the "dry drunk" very helpful. You may know someone who has managed to stop destroying their life by no longer indulging in alcoholic intoxication, but who is still irritable, depressed, hypercritical, and otherwise unhappy. Who would have thought that a problem this persistent could resolve with proper use of nutritional supplementation?

What could be called the corporate lie, that the purpose of life is acquisition of material wealth and power, is repeatedly exposed in <u>Natural Medicine</u>. Sociopathic by their very structure (the primary function is profit for the shareholder,) corporations have become an ever increasingly destructive force. Dr. Camo's caveat that "through a bizarre legal alchemy, corporations have now achieved the status of a human being," is balanced by an enlightened solution. Facilitating matriarchally-led, mutually supportive communities to supplant the old patriarchal hierarchical order provides encouragement to this otherwise desperate situation, enabling the healing first of ourselves and our families, and finally our planet.

To summarize, <u>Natural Medicine</u> provides a warning as to the threat to our health and our environment, the necessary information to start a healing process, and resources to proceed further.

Preface
By James Neubrander MD

It is common knowledge that in the enlightened age of the 21st century a new renaissance has begun and people are looking for alternative treatments to those offered by conventional medicine and pharmaceutical companies.

This is especially true when drugs have side effects or fail, and doctors are known to put Band-Aids on diseases but are not able to get most patients well. That is why this self-help book is perfect for those who have not been satisfied with the results they have obtained in the past and are eager to try some of the various types of natural, drug-free medicine that Dr. Camo has been practicing for over thirty years. You will find the "Dr. Camo" you meet within the pages of this book to be the loving, caring "Bonnie" that I have known and tremendously respected since we started working together in 1988 at the Brain Bio Center in Princeton, New Jersey. Bonnie was the physician who taught everything I knew about the subject at that time. With her we practiced Orthomolecular Psychiatry, as developed by Linus Pauling, Abram Hoffer, Humphrey Osmond, and our beloved mentor, Carl C. Pfeiffer (who rudely died on me only six months after I started working for him!) I am proud to say that we saved thousands of people diagnosed with mental illness from a life of institutionalization and dependence on neuroleptic drugs and their devastating side effects, by providing the specific nutrients that each of their individual brains needed in order to function properly.

After sixteen years at the Bio Center, in 1995 Dr. Camo was drawn to the field of homeopathy. At that time our paths split as I went on to specialize

14

in autism. Autism was a previously obscure disorder that affected only one in five to ten thousand children when Dr. Camo and I were in medical school. By the mid 90's it had become a national epidemic, and today it affects approximately one in one hundred children in America. There is no doubt in my mind that my experience under Dr. Camo's tutelage in the late 80's and 90's for sound nutrition has been an invaluable foundation to my success in treating children with autism, because all of them have extremely limited nutritionally-devoid diets. Though I do not practice homeopathy myself, my patients will attest to the fact that I am a firm believer in what it can do for patients. They will also attest to the fact that I frequently advise them to find a qualified homeopath in their quest to attain optimum health.

As you begin reading Dr. Camo's book, the first thing you will feel is the passion she has for what she does. By the end of the book, you will know that her *passion* is equally matched by her *compassion* for her patients. The book takes you on a journey that begins with the basics and ends with strong food for thought. Early on Bonnie will discuss the difference between real health-giving food as it occurs in nature, as compared to the imitation "food-like substances" that form a large part of the American diet, something that is contributing to the epidemic of obesity and chronic illness and the skyrocketing medical costs in America today. Importantly she is not a "back-to-nature nut" trying to "only sell her wares" by hiding the other side to nutritional debates, a good example being when she explains why some of us thrive on a vegetarian diet while others really need meat to be healthy.

It is interesting how Dr. Camo discusses the history of homeopathy from its origination two hundred years ago to how we understand it to work today.
In addition, it is quite commendable how Bonnie uses simple language to make this complex subject easy to understand. She covers everything from anxiety, anger and ADD, to First Aid, and how to help people recover emotionally and physically after natural disasters. She not only discusses the environment and health, she delves much deeper, explaining how these are affected by natural versus conventional approaches to the care

of our bodies. Toward the end of the book she speculates about our possible future evolution and how this may be affected by the choices we make today. In all well written books, the authors will include several testimonials written by patients who have benefited by the methods they are promoting. Dr. Camo's book is no exception to this, as she includes many enjoyable stories written in her patients' own words, describing how much they have benefited from her methods.

I thoroughly enjoyed the book and was enlightened by its content. I believe that it will have a similar effect on you. Enjoy~!

Introduction
How I Became a Homeopath

It seems my life was always unknowingly leading me to homeopathy. I grew up in Allentown, Pennsylvania, site of the first homeopathic school in America, the Allentown Academy, founded by Constantine Herring in the mid 1800's. He later moved to Philadelphia and founded Hahnemann Medical College, named after his mentor, the father of homeopathy, Samuel Hahnemann. By the time I graduated from Hahnemann as a medical doctor in 1978, it was totally allopathic, a regular medical school, where the ideas of its namesake were ridiculed.

I have been enamored of nature all my life, so I got a Bachelor of Science in Biology, then went for a Masters in Botany at the University of Pennsylvania. (I'm probably the only MD besides Andrew Weil with a background in botany.) I taught plant taxonomy at the U of P, collecting wild plants, drying and pressing them, then classifying them into the proper family and species, and learning all the Latin names. This knowledge was put to good use when I studied homeopathy, in which all plants as well as animals are known by their Latin names, the same all over the world.

I went to medical school with the intention of treating people with nutrition rather than drugs. After my internship in Internal Medicine in Allentown, PA, I moved with my family to New Jersey to work with Dr. Carl Pfeiffer at the Brain Bio Center near Princeton (later changed to Princeton Bio Center.) There we practiced Orthomolecular Psychiatry, treating mental illness with "megavitamin therapy". Pfeiffer did research on histamine as a brain neurotransmitter and devised protocols for different biochemical types of schizophrenia. We diagnosed and treated allergies, vitamin deficiencies, mineral imbalances, and heavy metal toxicities. This experience also facilitated the study of homeopathy, since most remedies are made from minerals and herbs.

I worked at the Princeton Bio Center for sixteen years, helping thousands of people control mental illness with daily doses of nutrients, individualized for each patient. Many people were able to get off or avoid being put on psychiatric drugs, and most were able to reduce their dosage, and live a freer, happier and more useful life.

The PBC relieved many people of mental as well as physical disorders, using nutritional principles. As I became more interested in homeopathy, I decided for various reasons to leave the Bio Center in 1995. I studied homeopathy intensively at the National Center for Homeopathy's Summer School near Washington DC, and then opened my practice integrating orthomolecular nutrition and homeopathy, which in my experience gives better results than using either method alone.

This book covers orthomolecular medicine, homeopathy, natural living, and other modalities I have learned and used over the past thirty years. Dr. Pfeiffer used to say that we were twenty years ahead of our time. Now, thirty years later, allopathic medicine, especially psychiatry, has still not caught up.

Homeopathy is a whole new way of looking at the world. Something containing no actual matter, only energy, enables people to cure their illness from the inside out. Modern physics now knows that the universe is not composed of matter, just concentrated probability waves of vibrating energy. Homeopathy was two hundred years ahead of its time.

Part 1

Natural Food

Chapter 1

The Truth about Fat and Carbs

The debate goes on about low carbohydrate versus low fat diets for health and weight loss.   Does fat make you fat? Or do carbs?   Why have Americans gotten fatter over the last forty years? Does it have anything to do with the low fat, high carb diet that was promoted by the United States government for many years, that familiar food pyramid with six to eleven carbohydrate servings at the bottom and a tiny triangle of fat and sugar at the top?

Dr. Robert Atkins was among the first to challenge this model in the 1970's with his high fat and protein, low carbohydrate diet. Many people did lose weight on it, but there were worries about the effects of all that fat on the heart.

According to a report at a recent Endocrinology Society meeting analyzing several controlled studies comparing low fat versus low carb diets, after six months, people on the low carb diet had lost twice as much weight, but by one year, the difference between the weights lost on the two diets was not statistically significant. (It didn't say whether the low fat people lost more later or the low carb people gained some back. The latter is more likely.)
Some people thrive on a high carb, low fat, mostly vegetarian diet such as those advocated by people like Nathan Pritikin and Dean Ornish, but it must be done wisely to avoid deficiencies of protein, good fats, and minerals like iron and zinc. People who tend to do well on this type of diet are those who are following their ethnic or ancestral diet, and those with type A or AB blood.

Atkins and low fat advocates like Pritikin and Ornish do agree on some things: avoid "bad" nutrient-depleted carbs like sugar, white flour, and corn syrup, (including "high fructose corn syrup" which appears on the label of most foods that come in boxes or cans). And avoid harmful unnatural fats like trans fats, which appear on labels as hydrogenated or partially hydrogenated oils.

Atkins did a good job of distinguishing among good and bad carbs by using the Glycemic Index (GI), a measure of how fast different foods turn to sugar in the body. Foods with a high GI, even some we think of as healthy, like brown rice, baked potato, and carrot juice, turn into sugar very quickly, causing release of a lot of insulin. The purpose of insulin is to remove excess sugar from the blood by allowing it to enter cells so it can be burned as energy. If there is too much sugar at one time, insulin, also known as the fat storage hormone, will turn most of it into fat and store it in the body. Atkins' diet and similar diets like the South Beach diet correctly recommend carbs with a low glycemic index like greens, salads, high fiber foods, and berries.

Where Atkins went wrong was saying all fat is OK, failing to differentiate among the health effects of saturated fats occurring naturally in meat and dairy products, artificially saturated vegetable fats, and the highly unsaturated fats in seafood.

Today there are many popular advancements on Atkins low carb diet, like Paleo and Ketogenic diets, and variations of fasting, which appear to be very helpful for controlling or even reversing disorders like Type 2 diabetes and even cancer.

Seafood is important for the essential fatty acids (EFA) needed by the brain and heart, the omega-3 fatty acids. Vegetarians can get their omega-3's from seeds like flax (linseed) and hemp seed, certain nuts (walnuts and butternuts), legumes, leafy greens, and omega-3 or DHA eggs. Many people may have difficulty converting short chain omega-3 found in plants to the long chain omega-3s needed by the heart and brain, so they may benefit from taking a supplement of fish oil, or perhaps even better, krill oil.

According to Udo Erasmus, <u>Fats that Heal, Fats that Kill</u>, people whose ancestors came from islands and coastal areas with a diet high in seafood may have lost the ability to convert the plant form of omega-3 (alpha linolenic acid) into the long chain form, docosahexaenoic acid (DHA) needed by the brain. This can only be gotten from seafood (including seaweeds). Populations affected may include northwest coast Native Americans, Inuit, Asian, Norwegian, Scottish, Welsh and Irish.

The question is not what the one best diet is for everyone, but which diets work best for which people. There is no one right diet for everyone, but there are diets that are bad for everyone, like the Standard American Diet (SAD), high in bad fats and bad carbs, thanks to the American food industry. What we need to learn is what are the good fats and good carbs, and how much of each is needed by each person, based on age, ethnicity and blood type.

Blood Type

The blood type "missing link" was discovered by Dr. James D'Adamo, a naturopath who used to put all his patients on a strict low fat vegetarian diet. Many improved on this, but some did poorly and got sicker. He tried to figure out why and started checking blood types. He found that in general, type A's, about forty percent of the population, thrived on vegetarian diets with protein from legumes and soy products, but did poorly on high protein diets with a lot of meat. Type O's, about half of the population, were just the opposite. They thrived on high protein and had high levels of stomach acid, needed to digest meat, and felt invigorated by intense physical activities.   All blood types were found to thrive on seafood, although type B's do better with fin fish than shellfish. B's and AB's were the only ones who really did well on milk products. Dr. D'Adamo published his research in 1980 in his book <u>One Man's Food</u>. The research was continued by his son Peter D'Adamo, who published <u>Eat Right 4 Your Type</u> in 1996.

Good and Bad Fats

Dr. Artemis Simopoulos, author of <u>The Omega Diet</u>, was a nutrition researcher for the National Institutes of Health (NIH). She grew up in Greece, a country with a "five-thousand year tradition of good nutrition", eating olives, fruits and vegetables that grew year round in the mild climate, eggs freshly laid by the family chickens, and "fish that had been swimming in the Mediterranean Sea only the day before". She came to the US in 1949 to attend Barnard College and found much of the food inedible: cottony white bread, rubbery cheese, and flavorless fruit.

She became a pediatrician and focused on infant and maternal nutrition. She gradually came to realize that many children with serious diseases had been "malnourished in the womb." This was then compounded by a poor diet lacking fruits and vegetables, but high in sugar, saturated fat, and margarine, with trans-fatty acids lurking everywhere. She organized the first international conference on essential fatty acids in 1985, and headed NIH research that showed that the human body functions most efficiently on a balanced one-to-one ratio of the two EFA families, omega-3 and omega-6. The American diet had become dangerously unbalanced, with up to twenty times as much omega-6 as omega-3. Most of the excess omega-6 was coming from vegetable oil.

Omega is the last letter of the Greek alphabet and is used in naming the different types of fatty acids. All fats are composed of one molecule of glycerin attached to three fatty acids, which are long chains of carbon atoms attached to hydrogen atoms. Saturated fats have every available chemical bond attached to a hydrogen atom, and are solid at room temperature, and not very active in the body. Unsaturated fats have certain spots which have less hydrogen and have two of the carbon atoms attached to each other by two bonds instead of one, forming a double bond. The double bonds allow for bending and flexibility of the fat molecules, allowing them to stay liquid at room temperature. The more double bonds, the colder the temperature at which fats or oils remain liquid (important for cold water fish). The problem with double bonds is that they are subject to being attacked by oxygen, making the oil rancid.

Monounsaturated oils like olive, canola and peanut oil have only one double bond and are very stable, not subject to oxidation and rancidity.

Polyunsaturated fatty acids (PUFA's) have more than one double bond. Omega-6 PUFAs have two. Omega-3's have 3 double bonds, starting 3 carbons from the "omega" end of the molecule (thus omega-3). Plants, animals and fish from cold, northern regions are composed of more highly unsaturated fats, because they need to stay flexible at low temperatures. The traditional food oils of northern Europe were flax and hemp seed oil, which are higher in omega-3 than the "southern" vegetable oils used today. Corn, safflower, and sunflower oils, which contain mostly omega-6, became available with modern processing methods in the 1950's and at first were thought to be healthy, at least better than the saturated fat in meat and butter.

Margarine was advertised as good for the heart, which has turned out to be a serious mistake. Margarine is made by starting with corn or other liquid vegetable oil and "hydrogenating" it until all the double bonds are saturated with hydrogen atoms, making it a solid, spreadable saturated fat, no healthier than butter. Actually it's worse than butter. Butter still has some bends in its molecules, but hydrogenated fat is in a "trans" form, with all of its atoms in a straight line, making it unable to fit into the cell membrane structures, and useless to the body. The body, being unable to metabolize this strange fat, stores it around the middle of the body, where it may remain forever, along with other toxic things in our food like pesticides.

Does the body hold on to fat to dilute the toxic chemicals it can't get rid of? Fat soluble pesticides end up in fat of animals (and those who eat the animals). Some pesticides have estrogen-like effects, disrupt our hormones and promote cancer. This is one of the reasons why high animal fat diets are associated with higher cancer rates. Another reason is that saturated animal fat, as well as excessive amounts of omega-6 oils, promote inflammation, now thought to be at the root of our most common chronic diseases like cancer, cardiovascular disease, and Alzheimer's disease. Omega-3's from fish and flax oil are anti-inflammatory and help prevent these conditions.

Chapter 2

Toxic Fat

In the last chapter, I asked the question, "Does the body hold on to fat to dilute the toxic fat-soluble chemicals it can't get rid of?" Is there a link between the American epidemic of obesity and chemical pollution of our air, water and earth? An article by Mark Hyman MD in the March/April 2007 issue of "Alternative Therapies" explores this hypothesis. He explains several key mechanisms by which toxins cause obesity.

Environmental toxins include chemicals and heavy metals. The heavy metals that cause the most health problems are lead, mercury, cadmium, arsenic, nickel, and aluminum. Chemical toxins include solvents and cleaning agents, prescription drugs, insecticides, herbicides and food additives. Mold toxins are a cause of sick building syndrome and other mysterious illnesses.

Organochlorine pesticides and polychlorinated biphenyls (PCB's) stored in body fat are released when body fat is used as fuel during a weight loss diet. These chemicals cause a decrease in thyroid hormone levels, lowering the metabolic rate and preventing further weight loss. Toxins also damage the mitochondria, the tiny powerhouses in cells, interfering with their ability to burn fat and create energy.

The liver has many enzyme systems for inactivating toxins and moving them out of the body. The ability to detoxify chemicals and remove heavy metals varies greatly among individuals. One protein called metallothionein is necessary for heavy metal detoxification. Mice bred without this protein gained more weight than normal mice. Metallothionein deficiency in humans is thought to be one of the factors in autism, in children who are genetically challenged at excreting heavy metals such as mercury, which was injected into them as the thimerosal preservative used in immunizinations given to infants and children in the 1990's, and still used in some vaccines today.

Toxins can also interfere with appetite-controlling substances in the brain, like leptin and alpha-MSH, causing hunger to increase. Children who were exposed to high levels of PCBs and DDE (a product of DDT) in breast milk, averaged twelve pounds heavier at puberty.

Fatty liver is the most common liver disease in America, affecting one in five. It is not caused by alcohol, drugs or viral hepatitis, but by excess sugar. Sugar, white flour and high fructose corn syrup are converted to triglycerides (fat) in liver cells. A fatty liver is unable to perform its job of detoxifying the body.

Removing Toxins

We can help remove toxins that cause obesity by eating organic foods, to avoid pesticides, hormones, and antibiotics. It is best to drink filtered water (rather than water in plastic bottles that will end up in a landfill forever – and who knows what harmful effect the plastic residues like phthalates have on us?) HEPA filters can be used to remove dust, molds and volatile organic compounds (VOC's) from the air, and shower filters to remove chlorine. Filling your house with certain houseplants helps clean the air. Heavy metal exposure can be reduced by avoiding aluminum pans and deodorants, lead paint, and tobacco, a major source of cadmium. Choose small fish like sardines, anchovies and wild salmon, rather than mercury-laden large fish like tuna and swordfish.

Encourage elimination of toxins by aiming for two bowel movements a day, drinking six to eight glasses of water a day, and working up a sweat by exercise, steam baths or saunas. "Depuration" is a treatment method used by practitioners of environmental medicine to treat chemical sensitivities and remove toxins, by means of low temperature saunas. Stretching exercises like yoga improve the flow of lymph and help flush out toxins. Eat detoxifying foods like cruciferous vegetables, dandelion greens, garlic, and berries. Drink green tea and herbal teas containing dandelion, ginger, licorice or cinnamon. High sulfur foods like eggs, whey protein, onions and broccoli provide sulfur-containing amino acids needed for detoxification. Season your food with herbs like cilantro, which helps remove heavy metals, and rosemary, containing carnosol which raises detoxification enzymes. Most fruits and vegetables tend to alkalinize the urine, which makes it easier to remove toxins.

Supplements that aid detoxification include a daily high potency multivitamin/mineral, vitamin C with bioflavonoids, milk thistle – an herb which benefits the liver, probiotics, omega-3 fatty acids, N-acetyl cysteine, alpha-lipoic acid, and L-carnitine. Zinc may be low in a vegetarian diet and may be supplemented to help displace heavy metals.

Chapter 3

Anti-Aging Food Rainbow

Colorful food is more nutritious! The colors that give beauty to flowers, vegetables and fruits are not only pleasing to look at, they are necessary for our health. The brighter the color, the more antioxidants! We need antioxidants to fight substances called "free radicals". These are not 1960's campus activists, but supercharged oxygen molecules that race around cells reacting with everything in sight. They damage DNA, cause mutations and cancer, inactivate enzymes, and destroy EFAs in cell membranes. This damage all adds up to produce aging. Antioxidants react with and "mop up" free radicals, to protect cells, and slow the aging process. Antioxidants come in all colors, including red lycopene, orange carotene, yellow lutein, green chlorophyll, blue anthocyanin, and purple resveratrol. Avoid colorless white food like sugar, flour, and white rice.

Lycopene

Lycopene is a red pigment found in tomatoes, especially cooked tomatoes. Since it is fat soluble, it is best absorbed with some fat, such as in tomato sauce containing olive oil, as it has been made in Italy for hundreds of years. (There were no tomatoes in Europe until after 1492, when Columbus "discovered" America.) When tomatoes were first brought to Europe, they were thought to be poisonous, like other members of the Nightshade plant family, deadly nightshade (Atropa belladonna), henbane (Hyoscyamus niger), and Jimson weed (Datura stramonium). Many of these poisonous plants have been made into valuable homeopathic remedies, as I'll discuss later.

The red tomato pigment lycopene, also found in watermelon, is a potent antioxidant that helps prevent cancer and heart disease. It helps prevent eye damage from free radical oxidation. It is very beneficial to the prostate gland and may reduce risk of prostate cancer and male sterility. A recent study in Europe showed that lycopene increased the body's natural killer (NK) cells by twenty-five percent in twelve weeks. NK cells are a part of the immune system that kills unwanted organisms and cancer cells in the body.

Another red antioxidant pigment is the recently discovered astaxanthin. It's what gives salmon, lobsters, crabs, and other shell fish, as well as flamingoes, their pink color.   Its antioxidant power is fifty times as strong as vitamin E. It is chemically related to lutein and zeaxanthin, but it works in both the fatty and watery portions of your cells, as a super-strong free radical quencher.

Carotenes

Beta carotene is an orange pigment found in carrots and in green, yellow and orange fruits and vegetables. It is the best known of a whole group of carotenoids that also includes alpha carotene, lutein and lycopene.   The carotenes aid in cancer prevention and are important for healthy eyes and skin. Beta carotene can be converted to vitamin A in the body, although this conversion may be difficult for people with hypothyroidism or diabetes. Cooking and pureeing carrots triples the amount of antioxidants that can be absorbed, compared to raw carrots. Leaving the skin on the carrots also increases availability of the antioxidants.

Lutein and Zeaxanthin

Yellow phytonutrients include lutein and zeaxanthin, both very important for maintaining the health of the eyes (as is astaxanthin), helping to prevent cataracts and macular degeneration. The macula, the point of sharpest vision in the eye, is yellow in color due to the presence of lutein and zeaxanthin. Lutein is a potent antioxidant that helps shield the lens and macula from free radical damage caused by years of exposure to oxygen and light. Lutein and zeaxanthin are thought to neutralize ultraviolet light and help filter out the dangerous short wavelength blue light, helping to maintain the photoreceptors and lining of the retina, (similar to the Ambervision and Blueblocker sunglasses that were popular a few years ago). Zeaxanthin also helps maintain the clarity of the lens, guarding against oxidative damage that results in cataracts.

Medical studies show that people who consume the most lutein and zeaxanthin are much less likely to develop age-related macular degeneration. Lutein also lowers the risk of heart disease and cancer. Lutein is found in broccoli, yellow corn, squash, and leafy green vegetables like spinach. Zeaxanthin is found in yellow corn, mangos, oranges, and egg yolks.

Chlorophyll

Chlorophyll, Greek for "green leaf", is another potential cancer blocker. Chlorophyll, of course, is the green pigment in plants that makes all life on earth possible. It is the basis of photosynthesis, the process by which plants use the energy of sunlight to convert carbon dioxide and water into glucose and oxygen. The glucose becomes plant matter, eaten by animals as food. All the oxygen that we breathe from the atmosphere was created by plants by the process of photosynthesis, using the green pigment chlorophyll. It is a curious fact that the chlorophyll molecule is exactly like the hemoglobin in our blood except that it contains magnesium instead of iron. Magnesium, so abundant in the chlorophyll of all green leaves, is one of the most commonly deficient nutrients, (especially in women). Magnesium deficiency is linked to chronic fatigue, anxiety, depression, insomnia, premenstrual syndrome (PMS), hypertension, heart arrhythmias, muscle cramps, and headaches.

Chlorophyll neutralizes dietary carcinogens, and protects cells from mutating in the presence of cancer causing agents. Broccoli and other members of the cabbage family have many sulfur-containing cancer-preventing compounds, including sulforaphane, dithiolthione, and isothiocyanates, which activate enzymes that detoxify carcinogens and carry them out of the cells.

Blue is for Berries

Blueberries, one of the few native North American fruits, are a powerhouse of nutrition. The United States Department of Agriculture

(USDA) Human Nutrition Center ranks blueberries number one, out of forty fresh fruits and vegetables tested for antioxidant activity. They have a wide range of powerful disease-fighting plant substances, known as phytochemicals. One of these, anthocyanin, produces their intense blue color, and is three times as powerful an antioxidant as vitamin C. Blueberries, and closely related bilberries, promote eye health, fight cancer, and help prevent kidney stones. Both blueberry and cranberry juice inhibit bacteria from sticking to the walls of the bladder, preventing urinary tract infections.

Blueberries and black currants have high concentrations of compounds that kill viruses and bacteria, such as E. coli, a common cause of gastrointestinal infections and diarrhea. In fact, black currants are an old folk remedy for diarrhea. Blueberries and other berries are high in antioxidants and anti-inflammatory substances that help protect the brain from free radical damage, and help prevent age-related memory loss. They help slow down and even reverse brain aging. The benefits in berries are packed within the smallest number of calories (for those counting). Even Atkins praised them. The antioxidant effect of blueberries is not harmed by freezing and storing, so, if you ever find them on sale or go berry picking, throw a few boxes in your freezer and savor them in muffins in the middle of winter.

Benefits of Red Wine

Resveratrol is a bioflavonoid antioxidant found in the skin of grapes. It is one of the active healthful ingredients in red wine. It helps to protect the heart and inhibit cancer formation. High levels are found in red wine, especially Pinot Noir, but there is very little in white wine. Red wine also contains even more potent antioxidants known as proanthocyanidins, from grape seeds, which dissolve in the alcohol of red wine during fermentation. They are not found in white wine, because the pulp, containing the seeds and skin, is removed from the juice immediately after the grapes are crushed. If you want the benefits of red wine without the alcohol, use it in cooking. The potent antioxidants in red wine may be the answer to the "French Paradox", explaining why the French seem to have less heart disease than would be expected, based on their high fat diet and high rate of smoking. Health-promoting red-purple pigments are also found in red and purple grapes, cherries, and berries.

Red wine also has antibacterial properties, not due to the alcohol, but due to polyphenols. The ancient Greeks poured wine into wounds as a battlefield antiseptic. (<u>The Food Pharmacy</u>, Jean Carper p. 306) Doctors in Nineteenth Century Europe noted that wine drinkers were more likely to survive cholera and typhoid epidemics, and advised mixing wine into water to help people survive these scourges. (Homeopathy users were also much more likely to survive these epidemics than those treated with conventional medicine.)

Chapter 4

The Pescivore's Dilemma

The fish-eater's dilemma is that the seafood diet, which is believed to have promoted expansion and evolution of the human brain, is now becoming too toxic to eat. The same omega-3 laden fish we have come to love for their nourishment of our brains are now burdened with brain-destroying dioxin, pesticides and mercury. Coal-burning power plants, which produce most of our electricity, release the mercury contained in coal high into the air with the smoke, where it is carried far and wide and deposited by rain on land and sea. Rivers carry it to the ocean where it is absorbed by plankton, which are eaten by fish. As big fish eat little fish, mercury builds up in the food chain. In large predatory fish like tuna and swordfish, the mercury and toxins far outweigh any benefit from their omega-3 content.

People who are able to thrive on a vegetarian diet are lucky, because it is much easier for them to find non-toxic, organic sources of food. They can get their omega-3 fatty acids from plant sources like flaxseed and flax oil, leafy greens and beans, in the form of alpha linolenic acid (ALA). Their bodies then convert the ALA into the long chain omega-3's, EPA and DHA, needed by the heart and brain. People whose ancestors have lived on seafood for thousands of years may have lost the enzymes needed for this conversion. As we get older, our bodies also become less efficient at this process, and we may have to eat fish, or take supplements of fish or krill oil, to maintain our health.
Another example of the loss of certain vital enzymes during the course of evolution is the inability of humans and other primates to produce vitamin C in our bodies, unlike almost all other animals that make as much vitamin C as they need. We lost the ability to produce vitamin C before we separated from other primates in our family tree, because our diet of fruit and leaves contained so much vitamin C that it was a waste of our metabolic energy to produce it. (Guinea pigs are also unable to produce

vitamin C. That is why they were chosen to be "guinea pigs" in nutritional experiments.)

Wild vs Farmed Fish

Salmon eat other fish, but don't live long enough to accumulate mercury. Wild Pacific or Alaskan salmon are a good choice for pescivores. All canned salmon is wild-caught, so far. They are not yet putting farmed salmon into cans. Canned pink salmon is still plentiful and inexpensive. Red salmon has more omega-3 and astaxanthin, and is more expensive. Atlantic salmon are raised in fish farms in the Pacific. Farm-raising a carnivorous fish like salmon is bad economics and bad ecology. It is a "protein sink". It takes two or three pounds of small wild fish to produce a pound of farm-raised salmon. It would be better for us and the earth to eat the small wild fish ourselves. Sardines, fresh or canned, are your best choice for health and the environment. They are tasty, loaded with omega-3 and the best food source of coenzyme Q-10. They are low in toxins, low on the food chain, and sustainably caught.

The idea of fish farms seemed like a good idea when it started out, but the crowded, confined fish, just like factory-farmed land animals, are prone to disease, so are fed antibiotics, as well as artificial coloring. The pink color of farmed salmon is an artificial pigment, to mimic the natural color of the antioxidant astaxanthin, which wild salmon get from eating tiny shrimp called krill. Fish farms spread disease and parasites that are wiping out the native Pacific salmon. Inland raising of plant-eating fish like tilapia makes a lot more sense.

Unlike fish farms, according to Taras Grescoe in <u>Bottom Feeders</u>, oyster farms are actually very beneficial to the environment. In areas like the Chesapeake Bay, these filter feeders clean the water by consuming excess nutrients washed from farmland, that would otherwise produce blooms of algae that eventually die and deplete oxygen, producing "dead zones", where nothing can live. But it may already be too late to save the Chesapeake Bay. Due to the proliferation of chicken factory farms around the Bay, as of the summer of 2011, the "dead zone" extended from

Baltimore Harbor to south of the Potomac River. A third of the once productive Chesapeake Bay is no longer capable of supporting sea life. Overfishing and pollution are rapidly depleting many fish that were once very abundant in the sea. If the fish disappear, will our brains deteriorate? Will society devolve into "Idiocracy", a movie I once saw about a society five hundred years in the future when everyone is stupid? Is this happening already? Spend a few hours watching television and you may think so.

Chapter 5

The China Study

<u>The China Study</u> is the most comprehensive study of nutrition ever conducted. The 2006 book, by T. Colin Campbell, describes his thirty-year study of dietary practices in different areas of China, correlated with rates of cancer, heart disease, and other disorders.   Campbell was raised on a farm and grew up eating lots of meat, milk and eggs. (He is now a vegetarian.) He went to veterinary school and then got a scholarship to do research in animal nutrition at Cornell. He studied toxic chemicals like dioxin and aflatoxin.

Protein's Dark Secret

He coordinated an investigation into the high rates of liver cancer in children in the Philippines. This type of cancer was thought to be due to aflatoxin, a carcinogenic toxin found in mold that grows on peanuts and grains. It was expected that malnourished children, deficient in protein, would have higher rates of cancer. The aim of the USAID project in the Philippines was to make sure that children got as much protein as possible. However, in this study, Campbell discovered a "dark secret." Children from the wealthiest families, who ate the most protein, had the highest incidence of liver cancer!

At the same time, he came across a relevant study from India, on rats. The rats were first given aflatoxin, and then one group was fed a twenty percent protein diet, and the other a five percent protein diet. Amazingly, every single rat on twenty percent protein developed liver cancer, and not a single one of those on five percent protein got cancer! This was a turning point in his career, contradicting everything he, and science in general, believed about protein and health.

Nutrition and Cancer

42

So he began his in-depth research into the role of nutrition in cancer, which was funded for twenty-seven years by the National Institutes for Health, the American Cancer Society, and the American Institute for Cancer Research. Studies on animals consistently showed that low protein diets inhibited initiation of cancer by carcinogens like aflatoxin. And if animals already had cancer, a low protein diet prevented it from growing. The effect of protein was so powerful, they could turn cancer growth on and off by adjusting the level of protein. Not all proteins were equally cancer-promoting. The worst was casein, which comprises eighty-seven percent of cow's milk protein. Protein from plants, like soy and wheat, did not promote cancer.

The China study covered sixty-five counties in rural China over a thirty-year period.   Blood samples and dietary information were collected from one hundred adults in each county. The study showed that people who ate the most animal protein had the most heart disease, cancer and diabetes. Cancer rates were higher in areas where vitamin C levels were low. Of course, these people in rural Chinese villages were not popping vitamin C pills. The vitamin C was coming mostly from fruit, and cancer rates were five to eight times higher in areas that ate the least fruit. Foods that are high in vitamin C, like fruits and vegetables, are also full of all the other colorful antioxidants that I have previously described. Vitamin C in the blood is a marker for all the other health-promoting antioxidants that were not measured. The bottom line, according to Campbell, is to get as much of your diet as possible from plants. Combining grains and legumes, like rice and soy products in China, provides complete protein, without increasing the risk of cancer and heart disease.

Is China Typical?

People with Type O blood reading this may be getting worried about how much the China study applies to them. According to Peter D'Adamo, <u>Eat Right for Your Type</u>, people with Type O blood are descended from hunters, and need red meat and vigorous exercise to feel strong.   There are fewer type O's in China, and more type A's and B's than in the US. Chinese people have been consuming their plant-based low-protein diet for thousands of years and are very well adapted to it, so that when more animal products began to be consumed by the wealthier classes, it might have had more of an adverse effect on them, than it would have had on populations that are adapted to a higher animal protein diet. Also, the source of casein, which had such a devastating cancer promoting effect on lab animals as well as children in the study, is cow's milk, which has never been a part of the traditional Chinese diet.

It is ironic that thousands of babies in China have gotten sick recently, and some have died, from melamine, a toxic substance put into milk to make it appear to have a higher protein level. As in the rest of the world, protein is still glorified in China even after the comprehensive study in that country showed a low protein diet to be healthier.

Chapter 6

Eating for A's

One of the best ways to improve effective brain power and academic performance is through proper diet. Whether you are a college student or a mother of school children, it is important to know how food affects the mind, mood, thinking and behavior.

Mood is definitely affected by food. Mood is dependent on neurotransmitters (NT's) such as serotonin and dopamine. Everybody knows about serotonin. It is the NT affected by antidepressant drugs called selective serotonin reuptake inhibitors (SSRI's), like Prozac™, Zoloft™, Paxil™, etc, which are commonly prescribed for depression. It is common knowledge that certain foods like milk and turkey are high in tryptophan, which produces serotonin in the brain, resulting in feelings of relaxation, contentment, and even drowsiness, especially in males. But the relaxed contentment after the turkey dinner may be due as much to the stuffing as the turkey.

Does Breakfast Make You Sleepy?

Although tryptophan is a component of protein, by a quirk of biochemistry, it is actually carbohydrates that cause serotonin levels to go up in the brain. A high carbohydrate meal, like the typical breakfast of cereal and milk, or toast with jelly and orange juice, is likely to make many children sleep through their morning classes. Eating carbs causes the pancreas to produce insulin, which transports amino acids other than tryptophan into the cells, leaving tryptophan free to cross into the brain where it is converted into serotonin.

A higher protein breakfast would be a better way for students to start their day. Eggs have been much maligned for their cholesterol content, but cholesterol is an essential component of body metabolism, needed to make sex hormones, and the adrenal hormones that we need to handle stress. Eggs contain "complete" protein, the amino acid ratios most perfectly matched to human requirements, as well as high levels of fat soluble vitamins A and D. If there is no time to cook and eat, hard boiled eggs can be made ahead of time and eaten on the way, or put in the lunch box. Eggs are one of the most important foods to buy organic rather than conventional, even though they may cost a little more. Pesticides end up in the fat of conventionally raised animals, and in their milk and eggs.

Another good choice is kids' favorite, the peanut butter sandwich. Use natural organic peanut or almond butter, not supermarket brands, and organic whole grain bread. (Conventionally grown peanuts have one of the highest levels of pesticides.) Nut butters are high in protein, unsaturated fat, B vitamins and minerals.

What about Tuna?

Tuna fish salad sandwiches are another mainstay of the brown bag lunch. Fish truly are brain food: high in omega-3 essential fatty acids, protein and zinc, but tuna are large predator fish, high on the food chain, full of mercury and other toxins. A better choice would be smaller fish like wild salmon and sardines. Not all kids like sardines, but canned salmon can be made into "tuna" salad that tastes as good as or better than the original. You can start with half tuna and half salmon, to get them used to the taste, if your kids are fussy.

My recipe for Salmon Salad:
One 14.75 oz can of Wild Alaska Pink Salmon (may contain bits of soft edible high-calcium bone which may be eaten)
1 organic onion and 1 stalk celery, chopped in food processor
4 organic hard-boiled eggs, chopped
1/4 cup mayonnaise
Blend all ingredients together.   Enjoy.

Chapter 7

Suppers for Sobriety

A few years ago, I attended the introductory meeting of a new group attempting to fill a "culture-wide void" in the area of long-term support for people with alcoholism and addictions. "Suppers for Sobriety" was created by Dorothy Mullen, co-founder of the Princeton Holistic Practitioners Exchange.   Dorothy has a Masters degree in alcohol and substance abuse counseling from The College of New Jersey, and found that this education, (like a medical school education), provided no information on nutritional and biological aspects of recovery. She wrote her Master's thesis on nutritional treatment of alcoholism and, comparing notes, we found that the research she based it on was pretty much the same as what I had used for a paper I presented to the National Council on Alcoholism in 1982. In other words, no significant research had been done on nutritional treatment of alcoholism in thirty years! (My paper: "Biotypes of Alcoholism", is presented as Appendix A.)

According to Dorothy, "Given a disease that is widely acknowledged to embrace the body, mind and spirit of the sufferer, the body has long taken a back seat to the mind aspect of addiction, has largely been characterized by medical intervention for detoxification, and pharmaceuticals for depression, anxiety, and symptom management."

Alcohol and Diabetes

Symptoms of vulnerability to alcoholism are the same as early signs of pre-diabetes, since they share biological roots related to insulin and blood sugar regulation. Most people in late stages of alcoholism are at least pre-diabetic and can no longer regulate blood sugar effectively. Many may have tended to hypoglycemia even before they began to drink. Even

48

after they have been abstinent, many suffer from the so-called "dry drunk syndrome", which has all the symptoms of low blood sugar. The coffee and cookies served at twelve-step recovery meetings are a set-up for relapse, and Alcoholics Anonymous has no opinion on outside matters, like nutrition.

Foods as Drugs

Many foods, especially fast foods, have drug-like effects. The insulin response to carbohydrates clears the blood of competing amino acids, so that tryptophan flows directly into the brain to produce the calming, mood-lifting serotonin. Many addictive foods and drinks, like coffee and alcohol, as well as tobacco, raise dopamine, producing mental alertness and energy. It is natural that recovering alcoholics are attracted to these substances, but they produce destabilization in the long run.
What is the solution? Slow food! Foods that stabilize blood sugar, supply the amino acids needed for neurotransmitter production, and provide basic good nutrition to relieve the screaming brain cells, and restore the poisoned liver enzyme systems that inactivate toxins and move them out of the body.

Therapeutic Friendship

Dorothy, who is also a gourmet cook and a master organic gardener, runs Suppers meetings for different groups several times a week in Princeton at lunch times and dinner times. Although she started with alcoholics because they are the most desperate, there are now also groups for diabetics, families of children with ADHD, people who want to lose weight, and just people who want to learn to cook healthy food, and enjoy the "therapeutic friendships" of cooking and eating together.

The greatest benefit and joy for me from the Suppers program has been the camaraderie of women working together to accomplish something for the benefit of all. Of course, men are welcome too, but there is a natural, feminine, cooperative energy reflected in the spirit and structure of the program. Everyone is encouraged to take a turn leading the opening blessing, or reading one of the concepts and boundaries before the shared meal. We are also encouraged to become facilitators, to learn the program and to start new Suppers groups in other locations, passing Suppers on in an organically growing movement. We are all valued for our roles as leaders and teachers.

This sort of non-hierarchical cooperative effort seems to come naturally to women, although it has been inhibited since the isolated nuclear family became the societal norm. In earlier times (and still existing to some extent in south Italy, where I now live), there were multigenerational extended families living together, grandmothers passing their culinary skills and traditions down to mothers and daughters. Now each woman struggles to feed her family, alone in her kitchen full of the latest modern conveniences, but no better the cook for all of the equipment. And many of us are exhausted after working all day at a paying job and – unsupported – we take the family out for fast food.

Female Bonding

Observing over the past three decades the kinds of stress that compromise our immune systems and rob us of our vitality, I've come to the conclusion that cooperative endeavors are very important for women's health. There are good reasons for this in terms of human evolution. Female bonding was particularly important in our early evolution, to ensure the survival of the young. Even though modern day babies are likely to grow to adulthood anyway, the wiring that makes women seek community and camaraderie has not gone away. We are still social creatures; we are designed to feel happiness and comfort in each other's company. Overwork, social isolation, and stress often result in depression, an indication that we are low in serotonin which is not – as some would have you believe - a Prozac deficiency. Helping and talking to each other are the antidote for such stress and isolation. They raise our serotonin levels and help us experience a sense of well-being that has been called a "Helper's High". Embracing our community and eating real food are much better ways to correct our unhappy mood chemistry. The alternative – stuffing ourselves with the carbohydrates we crave – is a less healthy, biochemical way of raising serotonin, yet so many of us reach for just that solution.

I was originally invited to Suppers for what I could contribute to the program design and literature. But I stayed because the nourishment of helping and working together was as important to my health as the wonderfully nourishing food we learned to prepare, to make us healthy "in body, mind and spirit."

The Family Table

Dorothy's rationale for creating a group based on "suppers" centers on two kinds of nourishment: 1) sound nutrition to repair a body ravaged by years of drinking or junk food eating, and 2) restoration of the family table, proven to be good prevention and an antidote to the isolation of addiction and recovery. She has trained many facilitators who are now running similar meetings in their homes and public locations around New Jersey.

Suppers groups focus on wholesome whole food preparation, stabilization of blood sugar through diet and exercise, and education about the various biological types of alcoholism and blood sugar regulation problems. For more information, please contact: www.dorothymullen.org, or www.TheSuppersPrograms.org "where people heal one meal at a time."

Chapter 8

The Real Mediterranean Diet

I visited Italy several times with my husband, who was born in Rome, before we decided to retire here, in south Italy. The everyday diet available to the average person here is much healthier than what most people eat in the United States. There are no "health food" stores, but food in regular stores may be comparable to health food here. Most produce, at least in the south, is grown on small near-by farms by traditional methods that don't rely on pesticides.   Genetically modified food is not allowed in Europe. Rather than have special "health food" for knowledgeable people, the aim is to have healthy food for everybody. Rather than take vitamins, they try to eat food that still contains nutrients. Although there are a few supermarkets in our town, most people shop in small stores, each specializing in one locally grown product like breads, cheeses, meat, fish, or fruits and vegetables.

Trebisacce by the Sea

We decided to settle in Trebisacce, a small town on the Ionian Sea, in the arch of the Italian "boot", near the town where my husband's father was born. On nearly every block there is a store selling dozens of varieties of extremely fresh fish (*pesce*), caught that day by local fishermen. One local specialty is *Rosa Marina*, tiny newborn fish less than an inch long, mixed with the hot peppers for which Calabria is world-famous.

Before buying our house here in Trebisacce, we used to stay at a small hotel called Parnasso. The hotel meals, prepared by a local woman, were simple, healthy and delicious. For lunch, vegetable and bean soup, then fresh fish and *sepie (*squid), lightly floured and sautéed in olive oil, followed by *insalate verde* (green salad) , finished with a bowl of fresh fruit, especially the locally grown small tangerines (*mandarini*) which were in season, and of course, grapes.

For breakfast, we would walk down the main street to the *"Bar Centrale"*. *Bar* in Italy doesn't have the same meaning as a bar here. They do serve wine and liqueurs, but mainly *caffé*. *Cappuccino* is only served in the morning. You can also get freshly squeezed juice (*spremuta*) from oranges grown near-by. They usually serve a glass of water to drink before your *caffé*, supposedly to clear your palate so the coffee tastes better. This is actually a good health practice, if you're going to drink coffee, since coffee is a strong diuretic.   *Caffé* in Italy is what we call *espresso*, a few tablespoons of very strong coffee in a tiny cup. It is expressed from the beans by steam, which releases the aromas. American style coffee is called *café lungo*, (long coffee). It is paradoxical that Italy, known for "slow food", drinks very fast coffee. A pot of tea is also available for tea lovers like me. With their morning *caffé*, most people will have a *"cornetto"*, a hot roll shaped like a trumpet (not to be confused with *"cornuto"*, which means something bad).

Slow Food

The main meal, which could be at noon or late evening, follows a definite order. First comes *antipasto* (before meal), which could be an assortment of fish, cheese or salami appetizers, olives etc. The *primo piato* is usually pasta, but could be *risotto* (rice), or *polenta* (cornmeal) in certain areas. You could also have a bean dish or vegetable soup as the "first plate". The *secondo* (second plate) is the main dish, meat or fish, served with *cortorno*, various vegetable dishes. Some of our favorites are *cicoria* (dandelion greens), and *carciofi* (artichokes). Delicious! After this there may be a plate of various local cheeses, walnuts, and always a bowl of fruits. Then *caffé*, perhaps with dessert, like *tiramisu* (which means "pull me up"), *pannecotto* "cooked cream", (like crème brulee or flan), or *gelato*, Italian ice cream, much more flavorful, yet with less fat and sugar than American ice cream. Wine and bottled mineral water are served with the meal. The wine is usually red, locally grown and delicious. The best wines are not exported, as they don't travel well.

The Culture of Olives

Many families have olive trees and grapevines in their backyard or at their parents' home in the country. In late fall the family gets together to pick the olives by hand, or by shaking them onto nets below. They are taken to the local olive press, where they are ground and pressed or centrifuged to separate the green-gold oil from the bitter watery juice of the raw olive. We picked two hundred pounds of olives by hand from the eight olive trees in our yard, which was pressed into twenty quarts of unbelievably delicious fresh, extra virgin oil, to use on our home grown salads.

The real Mediterranean diet, as I have experienced it, is way more than just pasta. I believe pasta for Italians has nostalgic value as the survival food that sustained Italy during the impoverished post-war period, along with beans, tomatoes, wild greens and olive oil. Those wild greens, once disparaged as "some weed the Italians eat" are now sold in the US in gourmet stores at fancy prices as *arugula, broccoli raab*, romaine lettuce, *radicchio*, and baby wild greens.

Chapter 9

Chocolate

Valentine's Day is an excuse for giving and eating chocolate, but no reason to feel guilty. Science has now shown that chocolate is actually very good for us. According to the *American Journal of Clinical Nutrition*, chocolate is an excellent source of antioxidant polyphenols, also found in red wine and tea. Polyphenols benefit the heart in several ways, such as preventing blood platelets from sticking together to cause blockages in blood vessels.   Studies at the University of California at Davis show that cocoa is a natural blood thinner, and a much tastier alternative to aspirin. Polyphenols also help prevent oxidation of low density lipoprotein (LDL), the so-called bad cholesterol, which contributes to heart attacks and strokes.

The best ways to enjoy chocolate's health benefits are in the form of hot cocoa, or semisweet dark chocolate. Milk chocolate doesn't have enough cocoa to be of any use, and is too high in sugar and fat. Look for brands such as El Rey™, Chocolove™, and Valrhona™, with at least seventy percent cocoa content. Half of a ninety gram (three ounce) bar will contain more than thirty grams of cocoa.

Chocolate and the Brain

Chocolate also contains many other compounds with interesting effects on the brain. The most studied are the methylxanthines, including small amounts of caffeine, and theobromine, a softer and more sensuous stimulant. The name theobromine, meaning "food of the gods," comes from Theobroma cacao, the Latin name for the cacao tree, source of cocoa. Despite the similarity of names, there is no relationship between cocoa, coca (source of cocaine), and coco, as in coconut.

Chocolate also contains phenylethylamine, or PEA, which stimulates the nervous system to release the brain's natural opium-like compounds known as endorphins. PEA floods the brain during orgasm and also when we are in love, producing that "giddy, restless feeling". Chocolate's reputation as an aphrodisiac goes back to the ancient Mayas and Aztecs, who raised it and used it extensively. The Aztec emperor Montezuma reportedly drank several goblets of cocoa drink before retiring with his harem. The Aztecs forbade women to drink it because of its aphrodisiac effects.   The legendary Italian womanizer Casanova also consumed chocolate before engaging in his favorite sport.

Chocolate Bliss

Another very interesting substance found in small amounts in chocolate is anandamide, named for the Sanskrit word for "inner bliss". Anandamide, discovered in 1991, is a chemical in the brain which has effects similar to substances found in marijuana. Anandamide is an endogenous cannabinoid, or endocannabinoid, part of the newest brain neurotransmitter (NT) system. Most of us have heard of NTs like dopamine, adrenaline, serotonin and melatonin. Anandamide is part of a whole other NT system, the newest, both in terms of its discovery, in 1991, and also probably in terms of our evolutionary development. Cannabinoid, of course, means cannabis-like, and cannabis does contain substances like tetrahydrocannabinol (THC), which fit the brain receptors designed for anandamide.   Anandamide produces a feeling of euphoria, which may explain the bliss some people experience when they eat chocolate.

Chocolate or Sex?

Chocolate is particularly loved by women. Fifty percent of women in one survey said they would choose chocolate over sex. In addition to the exotic chemicals in chocolate, the sugar triggers release of serotonin, which relieves anxiety and depression, and produces calmness. Even the fat in chocolate helps raise endorphins, relieving stress. Unlike many fats, the natural fat in chocolate, known as cocoa butter, does not raise cholesterol levels. The combination of fat with sugar in chocolate prevents the sugar from destabilizing blood sugar levels and causing hypoglycemia.

I don't recommend eating a lot of fat and sugar in general, but dark chocolate is one of the healthiest ways to eat them, in moderation, of course. One ounce a day, about a third of a chocolate bar, seems a reasonable amount. Always choose dark, bittersweet or semisweet over milk chocolate. Buy a small amount of really good, organic, sustainably raised, fairly traded chocolate from your health food coop, and enjoy enhancing your own health while you help save the world.

Part 2

Nutrients for Brain and Body

Chapter 10

Food and Mood Chemistry

Mood is definitely affected by food. Mood is dependent on neurotransmitters (NTs) such as serotonin and dopamine. Tryptophan is one of the twenty-two amino acids that make up the proteins in our diet, but our serotonin level is raised more by eating carbohydrates than protein. Carbohydrates are found in grains, breads, root veggies like potatoes and beets, sweets and fruits.
Women seem to crave starches and sweets more than men, probably because women tend to be lower in serotonin. Symptoms of low serotonin include: depression, anxiety, low self esteem, obsessive thoughts and behavior, seasonal affective disorder (winter blues), premenstrual syndrome, sensitivity to pain, craving for carbohydrates and alcohol, and recreational drug use. Serotonin is produced by the brain in sunlight. In darkness it is converted to melatonin, using up serotonin. That may be why women get hungry or crave cookies in the evening. Melatonin is the brain's natural sleep inducer.

Helper's High

A non-food way that women raise their serotonin levels and relieve depression is by talking to other women. Serotonin seems to be raised by sharing, talking, cooperating, and helping others, producing a "Helper's High". Serotonin levels go up in both the helper and the one who is helped. If this fact becomes widely appreciated, it could change the world!

Men usually have enough serotonin. They tend to be low in a different neurotransmitter, dopamine, found in meat. Ask men what they crave and they're likely to say meat. When men are depressed they are more likely to need dopamine than serotonin. Low dopamine depression is characterized by lethargy, apathy, lack of drive and motivation, and low sex drive.

Dopamine is raised by winning, being right, or making correct predictions. Predicting correctly is a useful skill in survival, rewarded by dopamine, the brain's pleasure chemical. Dopamine release is stimulated by all addictive drugs, including alcohol, cocaine and heroin. (But not marijuana, which has its own neurotransmitters, including anandamide, which hits the pleasure center, but not the addiction center of the brain). Even dopamine produced endogenously in the brain by winning or hope of winning can be addictive, as in compulsive gambling.

Brain Cats

Dopamine (DA) is converted in the brain to noradrenalin, also known as norepinephrine (NE) and then to epinephrine, better known as adrenalin. Adrenalin and NE are also produced in the adrenal glands, where they are responsible for the phenomenon of "fight or flight," the emergency reaction system discovered by Hans Selye. DA, NE, and adrenaline are collectively known as "catecholamines" or "Cats" for short. I like to think of DA as a pussycat, pleasurably lounging in the sun. NE is like a tiger, aggressively pursuing its prey, and adrenaline is a scaredy cat, fleeing from a dog.

When a person's NE level is too low, he may become depressed and apathetic, with low energy, drive, and focus, and poor concentration. He may be given a diagnosis of attention deficit disorder (ADD), but probably without hyperactivity. He may crave stimulation from carbohydrates, alcohol, coffee, or drugs like amphetamines and cocaine. This condition may be improved by taking the amino acid tyrosine in a dosage of 500 to 2000 mg one half hour before breakfast, mid-morning, and mid-afternoon. If there is insomnia, the afternoon dose may be skipped.

If NE is too high, the person may exhibit irritability, aggressiveness and hypertension. The amino acid gamma amino butyric acid (GABA), which is also a neurotransmitter, is an antidote to excess NE or adrenalin. The sublingual form can have an effect in minutes. I have seen it instantly calm a person in the midst of a panic attack (excess adrenalin). GABA goes straight to brain without cofactors. It may also lower high blood pressure. It also helps in withdrawal from benzodiazepine (Valium™ etc.) addiction. I have personally used it to help relieve back pain caused by excessive computer use.

Chapter 11

Brain Health and Longevity

The factors needed to maintain brain health are good food, certain nutritional supplements, exercise, brain exercise, and stress reduction. Protein is needed for amino acids to make neurotransmitters. Tyrosine, abundant in all protein foods, is the precursor of dopamine, noradrenalin, and adrenalin, the brain's natural "uppers". To stay alert, it's good to have some protein for breakfast and lunch.

Carbohydrates facilitate availability of tryptophan, the precursor to serotonin. Many people crave carbohydrates as a natural stress reliever. It is best to eat them in the evening to promote relaxation and sleep, but avoid refined sugar and white flour, which are devoid of nutrients and cause blood sugar imbalances. Use whole grains like brown rice along with legumes like beans, peas, and lentils to provide complete protein along with healthy, low glycemic carbohydrates.

Fat Heads

A very common cause of failing brain function is a deficiency of omega-3 fatty acids. The human brain is fifty percent fat, mostly docosahexaenoic acid (DHA), which the brain uses to build flexible cell membranes and synapses. DHA is best supplied by cold water oily fish like sardines, salmon, mackerel, and bluefish. Unnatural fats, like trans-fats found in hydrogenated oils, margarine, supermarket peanut butter, and most commercial baked goods, stiffen and gum-up cell membranes in the brain, heart and rest of the body, and should never be eaten. New labeling laws now require the amount of trans-fats to be listed, although they can get away with a certain minimum.

Vegetable oils like sunflower and safflower were once thought to be healthy, but are now known to be too high in omega-6. Olive oil is mostly omega-9, which does not promote inflammation and has some benefit for the heart and brain. It will not substitute for omega-3, but it will not cause harm like many vegetable oils which are high in omega-6. Fish oil supplements of omega-3 DHA and EPA may be beneficial, but there is no point in taking supplements with omega-6 and 9.

Brain Food

Fish really is brain food. According to the Aquatic Ape theory, it was a diet high in seafood that allowed our human brain to develop. Recent research has found supplementation with fish oil to be very effective in treating depression, including manic depression or bipolar disorder, and helping to prevent memory loss with aging. I have found this very useful in my own practice. Vegetarians can get omega-3 from flax oil and DHA supplements made from algae.

To maintain brain health throughout life, in addition to the right food, the brain will benefit from nutritional supplements, exercise, brain exercise, and stress reduction. Antioxidants are very important, and we get a lot of them from colorful fruits and vegetables. Another surprising big source is tea, which has been called "the thinking human's drink". (I was very glad to hear that, because I love tea.) Another surprise: black tea has more antioxidants than green tea, about eighty percent more, according to Jean Carper in <u>Your Miracle Brain</u>. Powdered tea mixes, and bottled tea drinks have little or none, and decaffeinated tea has half as much as regular black tea, according to Tufts University research. To help balance the caffeine, tea also contains L-theanine, which has a soothing, calming effect on the brain and has been called "instant Zen", useful for relieving stress and, taken in capsule form, promoting restful sleep.

Red wine in small doses, one glass a day for men, half a glass for women, helps prevent free radical damage and memory loss, and helps prevent strokes. Of course, too much alcohol kills brain cells. Like chocolate, a little goes a long way.

B Smart!

According to the Journal of the American Medical Association (JAMA), mild unrecognized vitamin deficiencies may cause subtle cognitive impairment in older adults. Mental functions like memory and problem solving were found to be directly correlated with blood levels of vitamin C and B vitamins like B6, folic acid and B12. People taking B vitamins scored better on tests of memory and abstract thinking. Studies at the University of Hawaii showed that elderly men who had taken vitamin C and E for years did better on cognitive tests. Research in Germany showed lower scores on mental tests in men and women over sixty-five who were low in any vitamin, especially C, B1, B2, and B12. They were also more likely to be depressed, anxious, angry, irritable, nervous and fatigued. As a precaution, everyone should take a good, high potency multi-vitamin/mineral and perhaps extra B's (50 mg) and C (500 to 2000mg per day).

Vitamin B6 is especially important for the brain. It is required for the synthesis of neurotransmitters like serotonin, dopamine and GABA. Along with B12 and folate, B6 reduces homocysteine, which damages the heart and brain. B6 helps convert body stores of carbohydrate into glucose, the brain's major fuel.

The Sunshine Vitamin

Vitamin D has been recognized as a potent fat soluble antioxidant, even more powerful than vitamin E. Deficiencies of D have been found in Parkinson's and Alzheimer's disease. Four hundred international units (IU) was always thought to be adequate, but recent studies show that we may need 1000 or 2000 IU or more, especially in winter, when we can not benefit from free vitamin D from the sun. D3 is the most effective form to take as a supplement.

Natural Cholesterol Control

Coenzyme Q-10 is needed for energy production in the mitochondria, tiny "spark plugs" in every cell where conversion of food into adenosine triphosphate (ATP), the chemical energy that fuels life, actually takes place. Co Q-10 also works with vitamin E to prevent "lipid peroxidation", destruction by free radicals of the liquid fats that make up half of the brain. Co Q-10 also regenerates depleted vitamin E. Statin drugs prescribed to lower cholesterol cause depletion of CoQ-10, so be sure to take Co Q-10 (30 to 100 mg per day) if you are taking these drugs. Better ways of lowering cholesterol include taking vitamin B3, also known as niacin, (use the "no flush" form to avoid the harmless temporary skin redness and heat caused by regular niacin, although some people do enjoy the flush). Fish oil, 2000-4000 mg per day, also helps lower cholesterol as well as triglycerides, in addition to its many other benefits to the brain.

AGES

Perhaps the most important and overlooked brain antioxidant is alpha lipoic acid (ALA). Unlike most other antioxidants, it is soluble in both fat and water. It easily passes through the "blood brain barrier" and goes directly to brain cells under attack. It is the only antioxidant that can regenerate itself as well as other used-up antioxidants, such as vitamins C, E, coenzyme Q-10 and glutathione. It also helps block production of sugar-damaged proteins called advanced glycation end products (AGES), which, as their name implies, do age you. ALA helps prevent and treat strokes and diabetic neuropathy. The recommended amount is 200 to 600 mg a day.

Memory lapses and slower recall of names and words are not necessarily signs of impending Alzheimer's disease. Depression, hypothyroidism, and nutritional deficiencies should be ruled out before imposing ominous diagnoses. Older people have reasons to be depressed, due to losses in their lives, of spouses, friends, abilities and resources. However, recent studies indicate surprisingly that people in their sixties are less depressed than people in their forties and fifties, and they become less depressed the older they get.

Vitamin B12 deficiency is very common in older people, causing symptoms like depression, anxiety, memory gaps, and confusion. B12 occurs only in animal products and requires stomach acid for absorption. Older people tend to have lower levels of stomach acid and digestive enzymes. People on acid blocking drugs or proton pump inhibitors (PPIs) for gastro-esophageal reflux disease (GERD) are also at risk for deficiency of B12, as well as minerals that require acid for absorption. Vegetarians and vegans get a lot of folate from fruits and vegetables, which could mask a B12 deficiency on a blood test.   B12 supplements should be taken in sublingual form, dissolved under the tongue for direct absorption into the bloodstream, bypassing the gastrointestinal tract.

Zinc and the Brain

Zinc is one of the most important minerals for the brain, needed for synthesis of neurotransmitters, and for growth and repair of brain and body. Zinc is abundant in seafood, and may need to be supplemented by vegetarians. Zinc requires stomach acid or vitamin C for absorption. Zinc helps displace harmful heavy metals like lead, cadmium and mercury. Older people may have high levels of lead, which we absorbed from the environment before lead was removed from gasoline, and high mercury from dental amalgams most of my generation had put into our teeth as children. Lead is a neurotoxin that causes depression, insomnia, and poor memory.

Mercury and the Mind

Seafood is a good source of zinc and omega-3 good fats, but unfortunately, now is also a big source of toxic mercury. Symptoms of mercury poisoning, according to Alan Schmukler in <u>Homeopathy, the Home Handbook for Survival</u>, include memory loss, shyness, timidity, loss of will power, indecision, lack of confidence, apathy, suicidal thoughts and violent impulses. Many common diseases of aging like Alzheimer's, hormonal imbalances like hypothyroidism, autoimmune disorders, chronic fatigue, fibromyalgia, and psychological problems as listed above are now thought to be at least partly related to mercury and other toxic heavy metals.

Mercury released from burning coal in power plants falls in rain on land and water, ending up in rivers, lakes, and finally the sea.   It enters the food chain, increasing in concentration as big fish eat little fish, ending up at the highest levels at the top of the food chain: whales, polar bears, and us. (Another reason to promote renewable, non fossil fuel energy sources like wind, and solar power.)

Grow New Brain Cells

It used to be thought that we were born with all the brain cells we would ever have, that brain cells (neurons) were unable to divide and multiply like other cells in the body. It is now known that the brain is capable of growing new neurons throughout life, even in old age. Physical exercise is one thing that increases this neurogenesis. The brain also grows new neurons when it learns or experiences something new. Using skills we have already mastered brings comfort, but doesn't make the brain grow. The mental decline many people experience as we grow older is not mainly due to death of nerve cells, but may be due to loss and thinning out of dendrites, nerve cell branches that connect with other neurons. It is now known that old neurons, when stimulated by novelty, can grow new dendrites to compensate for losses.

Brain exercise called Neurobics (described in <u>Keep Your Brain Alive</u>, by Katz and Rubin) stimulate the brain with nonroutine ways of using the various senses: vision, hearing, smell, taste and touch. The brain is hungry for novelty. Try breaking routine by getting dressed or showering with your eyes closed, taking a different route to work, or shopping at a farmers market instead of the supermarket. Combine senses, such as listening to a particular song while smelling a specific aroma. Use your sense of touch instead of vision to find the right key to open your door. Experiment with novel cuisines from other countries. Try eating with chopsticks. Start a new hobby. Learn a new language, a musical instrument, or how to use a smartphone. Any of these will stimulate the brain to grow new neurons and make new connections between neurons, keeping your brain young and healthy.

Chapter 12

Natural Treatment for Depression and Bipolar Disorder

The currently popular theory is that depression is caused by a lack of serotonin. It is supposed that SSRI (selective serotonin reuptake inhibitor) antidepressants work by blocking "reuptake" of unused serotonin back into the neuron, so more stays in the synapse, making connections with other neurons. If this is true, it could backfire in several ways.   With more serotonin around, the neurons would need fewer receptors to pick it up, resulting in "down-regulation" or destruction of "excess" serotonin receptors. If the drug is stopped, the patient is left with fewer serotonin receptors, so depression may return, even worse than before. Also, since neurons can no longer collect and reuse serotonin, it eventually becomes depleted. It's like whipping a tired horse.

If depression is due to low serotonin, (which psychiatrists never test for; they just assume), it may be related to a deficiency of something needed by the brain, like vitamin B6, which is a cofactor required for production of serotonin from its precursor, tryptophan, an amino acid found in all protein food.

The Tryptophan Saga

Forty years ago, my colleagues and I at the Princeton Brain Bio Center, and other nutrition-oriented physicians, treated depression, particularly the anxious, agitated type, with tryptophan, (also known as L-tryptophan), which was then available over the counter. It was very effective for depression, anxiety, insomnia and many other problems. In 1989, a mysterious illness arose which made hundreds of people ill, and caused a few deaths. The US Center for Disease Control (CDC), linked this

Eosinophilia-myalgia syndrome to tryptophan, and all tryptophan was pulled from the market. It was subsequently discovered that the illness was only caused by tryptophan from a Japanese company, Showa Denko, which used genetically-engineered bacteria in the production process, resulting in a toxic contaminant. Still, tryptophan was not allowed back on to health food store shelves for sixteen years, although it eventually became available from compounding pharmacies, with a doctor's prescription, and is now finally available again in health food stores. By a strange coincidence, the natural antidepressant tryptophan, which raises serotonin, was outlawed in the same year that serotonin-stimulating antidepressants, SSRIs, were introduced. When wondering why certain things happen, it is often useful to ask yourself, "Is it an accident? Who benefits?"

Do Antidepressants Work?

Antidepressants are now the most commonly prescribed category of drug in the United States, with more than a quarter of a billion prescriptions written in 2007, at a cost of $11.9 billion. After twenty years of use, many recent studies indicate that these drugs don't even work! Several articles in allopathic (conventional) medical journals in the past few years indicate that SSRI antidepressants are virtually nothing more than placebos. These studies have received little notice in the United States, but have stirred up major controversy in Europe.

A study published in the <u>Public Library of Science Medicine Journal</u> in February, 2008, by Irving Kirsh, PhD, Brett Deacon, PhD, et al, analyzed the raw data presented to the FDA, of thirty-five clinical trials of fluoxitine (Prozac), paroxitine (Paxil), venlafaxine (Effexor) and nefazodone. A meta-analysis of these studies showed no significant difference between drug and placebo in patients who were moderately or severely depressed. Only in patients who were extremely severely depressed was there a slight difference, and this was not because of a response to the drug, but because of a decreased response to the placebo.

A January 2007 article in the <u>New England Journal of Medicine</u> by Erick Turner MD showed that medical journals mainly publish only articles that show a positive effect in an antidepressant drug trial. Of seventy-four studies filed with the FDA, thirty-seven of thirty-eight positive trials were published, while only eight of twenty-four studies showing no effect were published. The rest were quietly "shelved". Dr Turner also showed that the same positive studies were often published multiple times in slightly different forms.

An April 2000 meta-analysis by Arif Kahn MD, published in the <u>Archives of General Psychiatry</u>, showed that more depressed patients on anti-depressants committed suicide than those on placebo.   There is now a black-box suicide warning on SSRI packages.

Omega-3 for Depression

Depression is commonly caused by nutritional deficiencies, particularly of essential fatty acids. Since the brain is fifty percent fat, we are really all "fatheads", but not just any fat will do. As your mother told you, fish really is brain food. The Aquatic Ape theory of human evolution hypothesizes that it was a diet high in seafood that allowed our human brain to develop. Recent research has found supplementation with fish oil very effective in treating depression, including manic depression or bipolar disorder.

The first study of omega-3 fatty acids in psychiatric disorders was published in 1981 by Donald O. Rudin of the Eastern Pennsylvania Psychiatric Institute (EPPI) in Philadelphia. He used high doses of flax oil, a major source of a short-chain omega-3 fatty acid called alpha linolenic acid, or ALA. Some patients with bipolar disorder developed mania, hypomania, or rapid mood shifts on ALA. The doses in this first study were much higher than what is recommended today, and the preferred source is now fish oil, which contains the long chain omega-3's, EPA and DHA, found in the human brain.

Rudin's book, <u>The Omega-3 Phenomenon</u>, published in 1987, describes what he calls the "modernization disease syndrome" (MDS), a lipid deficiency/toxicity syndrome responsible for a host of diseases that became rampant in the Twentieth Century. Heart disease, strokes, diabetes, obesity, and cancer became the leading killers, while arthritis, digestive disorders, anxiety, depression, attention deficit/ hyperactivity and schizophrenia also greatly increased.

Rudin relates these modern epidemics to the missing link, omega-3 fatty acids, which was overlooked in the usual nutrition experiments based on rats and mice, because these rodents don't require the brain-building nutrients needed by primates. Monkeys on a laboratory diet with corn oil as the only fat developed dermatitis, dandruff, diarrhea, and dementia, which were relieved within two months after adding flax oil.

Andrew Stoll MD, in <u>The Omega-3 Connection</u>, published in 2001, describes his studies of patients with treatment-resistant major depression. These patients had not responded to treatment with any conventional antidepressants, but when fish oil was added, even the patients were surprised at their improvement. This makes sense because without omega-3 fatty acids, the brain cannot function normally, so even the strongest antidepressant will be ineffective.

He then went on to studies of patients with bipolar disorder. In 1997 he presented the results of a planned nine-month double-blind placebo-controlled study of thirty high-risk patients with bipolar disorder, treated with fish oil. A four month preliminary analysis of the data showed such amazing results with fish oil compared to patients on placebo, who were no better or even getting worse, that he cut the study short and offered fish oil to all participants, and published the results in the <u>Archives of General Psychiatry</u>. In the bipolar study, he gave patients 9.6 grams of omega-3 per day, (6.2 of EPA and 3.4 of DHA), but he finds that in clinical practice, 2 to 5 grams per day is adequate for most patients.

Thyroid and Depression

Hormonal imbalances are another very common cause of depression. I have seen many patients, especially women, who had all the signs and symptoms of hypothyroidism: depression, fatigue, weight gain, hair loss, dry skin, low body temperature, and high cholesterol. But their blood tests for thyroid function were "normal". They had been to many doctors who seemed to look only at the numbers, rather than the person, and refused to treat them for a condition that seemed obvious when you actually looked at and listened to the patient. Many patients have been given a new life with inexpensive natural thyroid hormone or supplements like tyrosine and sources of iodine like kelp and other seaweeds, which the body needs to make thyroid hormones.

Most doctors test for thyroid problems by getting only a TSH (thyroid stimulating hormone) level. TSH is a hormone produced by the pituitary gland, to stimulate the thyroid to produce its hormone thyroxin, also known as T4. If the thyroid is sluggish in its production of T4, the pituitary sends more TSH to whip it into action, so a high TSH level actually indicates a low-functioning thyroid. A low TSH, on the other hand, is generally considered indicative of an overactive thyroid, or taking too much thyroid medication. But a low TSH could also mean that the pituitary is incapable of producing adequate TSH. A T4 level can be done to distinguish between these conditions. In either case, the treatment is usually prescription of a synthetic thyroid hormone containing only T4. I got better results using desiccated thyroid, made from animal glands, containing both T4 and T3.

Hypothyroidism may also be caused by Hashimoto's thyroiditis, an autoimmune disorder. This can be diagnosed by lab tests for thyroid antibodies. A T3 level should also be done. T4 is the main circulating thyroid hormone in the bloodstream, but in order for it to become active, it must be converted into T3, triiodothyronine. Many people are incapable of making this conversion, particularly people whose ancestors underwent periods of famine and starvation. The thyroid hormones control the rate of body metabolism, or burning food to produce heat and energy. When little food is available, the body can shift into conservation mode, burning less fuel in order to conserve energy and survive. The body accomplishes this by converting less T4 into T3. When more food becomes available, the body is supposed to shift back into making more T3 and increasing available energy, but sometimes it gets stuck in the low energy conservation mode. This also happens to people who go on a low calorie diet to lose weight. They may lose weight at first, but then the body thinks it's starving and shifts into conservation mode, so they have no energy, and gain weight on fewer calories than they were able to burn before dieting.

One way to overcome this is to eat more, high quality nutritious food, and get more exercise, which raises body temperature and burns calories. A thyroid supplement may also be needed. One way of testing for low thyroid function is the Broda Barnes method. Low body temperature is a major indicator of low thyroid function. Normal oral temperature is 98.6 degrees Fahrenheit (37 Celsius). I have treated many patients with temperatures of 96 to 97 degrees, who benefited greatly from thyroid treatment. Dr. Barnes recommended taking your own temperature by putting a thermometer under the arm for ten minutes on waking, before getting out of bed. An axillary temperature of less than 97.8 degrees may indicate hypothyroidism.

Adrenal Fatigue

Depression with chronic fatigue may also be due to low adrenal function, which often begins after unremitting stress that burns out adrenal reserves, or from chronic exposure to toxins like heavy metals. Mercury can lower both adrenal and thyroid function. Adrenal insufficiency is now easy to detect through a saliva test, and easily treated with low physiological doses of natural cortisol and/or supplements like pantothenic acid, vitamin C, B6, and zinc, or the adrenal hormone precursors dehydroepiandrosterone (DHEA) and pregnenolone, as well as adaptogenic herbs like ginseng and ashwaganda.

Grief is Normal

Causes of depression include "exogenous", due to outside factors, and "endogenous", due to factors within your mind or body. Exogenous depression, such as sadness and grief due to loss of a loved one, is a normal condition, as your mind comes to terms with its new situation. This is not a time for prescription of antidepressants, which may change a normal condition into a drug dependency. I never find instructions in the PDR (Physicians' Desk Reference, which gives information on all prescription drugs) for how to get a patient off a drug, only how to get them on. I guess they assume, and hope, you'll be on it forever.

Chapter 13

Orthomolecular Psychiatry for Schizophrenia

The term orthomolecular psychiatry was coined by Linus Pauling (winner of two Nobel prizes, for chemistry and peace) in his famous article in <u>Science</u> magazine in 1968. It refers to the treatment of mental illness with substances that occur naturally in the human body, such as vitamins, minerals, amino acids and essential fatty acids. The brain is dependent on nutrients supplied by the body. If these are inadequate due to a poor diet (deficiency) or a genetic need for more than the usual amount of a particular nutrient (dependency), the brain may be unable to function normally.

In the early decades of the Twentieth Century, mental hospitals in the southern United States were filled with people suffering from a schizophrenia-like syndrome called pellagra. It was discovered that this condition was caused by a deficiency of the B vitamin niacin, due to a poor diet of corn and fatback. Corn is very low in niacin as well as tryptophan, from which the body can make niacin.   In the early 1950's two psychiatrists in Saskatchewan, Canada, began treating schizophrenics with large doses of niacin, and had great success. Abram Hoffer MD, PhD and Humphrey Osmond, MRCS, DPM, conducted the first double blind tests in the field of psychiatry, using at least one gram each of niacin and vitamin C three times a day.   Many patients showed great improvement, being able to work and stay out of the hospital. Hoffer's criterion for whether a patient had recovered was that he was able to work and pay taxes.

It's Psychedelic!

Dr. Osmond was also the originator of the term "psychedelic", meaning mind-manifesting. Lysergic acid diethylamide (LSD) had recently been discovered by chemist Dr. Albert Hofmann at Sandoz pharmaceutical company in Switzerland, in 1943. Drs. Hoffer and Osmond experimented with using it to produce an artificial psychosis, in order to learn how to better treat schizophrenics. (This was before LSD was promoted by Harvard professor Timothy Leary and became popular among the Hippies in the 1960's.) Dr. Osmond discussed his research in correspondence with Aldous Huxley, in 1956. They were trying to come up with a neutral name to describe this sort of drug, to replace terms like hallucinogenic and psychotomimetic. Huxley wrote to Osmond, suggesting "phanerothyme", meaning soul-manifesting, with the couplet:

> To make this trivial world sublime,
> Take half a gramme of phanerothyme.

Osmond wrote back with his suggestion:

> To fathom hell or soar angelic,
> Just take a pinch of psychedelic.

He had no idea how widely this term would come to be used.

Tranquilizer Drugs

Shortly after Hoffer and Osmond's study, the first neuroleptic tranquilizer, Thorazine™, was introduced to North America in 1953, and promoted aggressively by psychiatrists and pharmaceutical companies. These antipsychotic drugs are thought to work by blocking dopamine, known as the brain's pleasure chemical. Dopamine in the cerebral cortex allows you to make connections, solve puzzles, and form a whole picture from incomplete data. In excess, it could make everything fit together too well, producing paranoia, where the whole world is conspiring against you. (But remember, just because you're paranoid doesn't mean they're not out to get you!)

Side Effects of Drugs

Dopamine also works in deep brain structures called the basal ganglia, to coordinate body movements. Conventional neuroleptics also block dopamine here, resulting in an incurable movement disorder known as tardive dyskinesia (TD), resembling Parkinson's disease. Unknown to conventional psychiatrists, TD can be prevented by certain vitamins and minerals, including dimethylaminoethanol (DMAE), a form of choline, and the mineral manganese. In thirty years of treating schizophrenic patients with megavitamins, I never had anyone develop tardive dyskinesia, even if they were also on neuroleptic tranquilizers.

Toxic Psychiatry

The new generation of "atypical" antipsychotics, such as Clozaril™, Zyprexa™, Seroquel™, and Risperdal™, are less likely to produce movement disorders, but they cause other problems, including obesity and diabetes. According to Peter Breggin, in <u>Toxic Psychiatry</u>, since these drugs do not produce tardive dyskinesia, psychiatrists are lulled into believing that they are relatively harmless to the brain, and give them in higher and higher doses. But they may cause tardive dementia and tardive psychosis, the word "tardive" meaning that symptoms persist and even get worse when the drug is withdrawn. It is very difficult to withdraw patients from these drugs, yet their mental functions may be deteriorating the longer they stay on them.

According to Eva Edelman, <u>Natural Healing for Schizophrenia</u>, "Psychiatric drugs have the potential to induce a supersensitivity psychosis in the world's sanest human, forcing the individual into a lifelong drug dependency." Blocked dopamine synapses become hypersensitive, so when the drug is withdrawn, paranoia and hallucinations become worse than ever. Once the patient is on orthomolecular therapy, an attempt can be made to withdraw the drugs very gradually, but many patients will need to stay on a small dose, as the brain has become dependent on it. The natural psychosis has become a "tranquilizer psychosis", as Dr. Hoffer calls it.

Psychiatric diagnostic labels are not based on the cause of the problem, but merely on a catalog of symptoms, as listed in the Diagnostic and Statistical Manual (DSM), the Bible of psychiatry. Orthomolecular psychiatry attempts to determine the biochemical cause of the brain malfunction and treat it with the appropriate nutrients.

Histamine and the Brain

According to the research of Dr. Carl C Pfeiffer, at the New Jersey Neuropsychiatric Institute in the 1970's, the majority of schizophrenics suffer from a deficiency of the brain neurotransmitter histamine, a condition he named "histapenia". You may be familiar with histamine as that nasty substance that causes allergy symptoms and asthma, as well as acid reflux, for which you take various kinds of antihistamines and histamine blockers. Histamine is released from white blood cells called basophils in response to allergens.

Dr. Pfeiffer was one of the first to realize that histamine was also a neurotransmitter, a chemical messenger in the brain, in fact perhaps controlling other neurotransmitters like dopamine and serotonin. One of the actions of tetrahydrocannabinol (THC), the best known constituent of marijuana, is to decrease histamine levels in the brain. This property is probably responsible for marijuana's historical use as a treatment for asthma.   The small percentage of people who become paranoid on marijuana (when it is not due to the realization that they could be arrested and put in jail for performing an illegal act), are probably histapenic. Not all people with low histamine are schizophrenic, but histapenics may occasionally develop paranoid symptoms on other substances that block histamine, like ulcer and acid reflux drugs.

Dr. Pfeiffer discovered how to treat schizophrenia with vitamin B12, folic acid, and niacin, which raise histamine. He found that many patients had excessive copper, which lowers histamine. At the Brain BioCenter, we used zinc and vitamin C to remove excess copper, as well as heavy metals like lead, cadmium and mercury.

Dr. Pfeiffer's research showed that about ten percent of people diagnosed with schizophrenia actually had the opposite condition, too much histamine, which he called "histadelia". These people would probably be diagnosed today as bipolar or schizoaffective. High histamine is generally associated with conditions like chronic depression, bipolar disorder, suicidal tendencies, chronic alcoholism, and obsessive compulsive disorder (OCD), as well as allergic conditions. Histadelia can be treated with methionine, an amino acid, which detoxifies histamine by methylation. SAMe (s-adenosyl methionine), a new and effective treatment for depression (as well as arthritis) is a derivative of methionine.

Pyroluria

Pfeiffer found that many schizophrenics and some normal people under stress have pyrolles in their urine, which combine with zinc and vitamin B6, causing these nutrients to be lost in the urine, a condition known as "pyroluria". This type of schizophrenia tends to run in families and can be precipitated by stress.   Common symptoms include changes in sensory perception (disperceptions), intolerance to some protein foods, alcohol, or drugs, morning nausea, lack of dream recall, white spots on fingernails, stretch marks, inability to tan, irregular periods, abdominal pain and constipation. Any of these may be worsened by stress. Pfeiffer speculated that pyroluria was the cause of the mysterious lifelong disability suffered by Charles Darwin, discoverer of evolution by natural selection. He also thought that the poet Emily Dickenson suffered from this condition.

Pyroluria quickly responds to high doses of vitamin B6 and zinc. Zinc is abundant in meat, fish and shellfish. Oysters have more zinc than any other food, which may be the reason for their reputation as an aphrodisiac. Zinc is required for the prostate, sexual function and testosterone production. The old idea that masturbation causes blindness or madness could have some basis in truth for a zinc-deficient adolescent,

84

since about one milligram of zinc is lost in each ejaculation. I
wonder if this has anything to with the reported loss of vision in men taking
Viagra™. The erectile dysfunction for which they're taking Viagra could be
due to lack of zinc, which is exacerbated by the increased sexual activity.
Zinc is very important for the eyes, and deficiency may contribute to
macular degeneration. Vegans should be aware that it is difficult to get
enough zinc on a totally vegetarian diet, and they may need to take a
supplement.

MS's Story – schizophrenia
*I had a normal life until I was sixteen, but then everything changed. I felt
depressed and paranoid and was later hospitalized with a feeling of
mania. This first episode was written up as a psychotic episode and
Haldol was prescribed and taken for the following two months.
Six months later I became manic, was hospitalized, and took Mellaril and
Lithium. I was then diagnosed bi-polar. I took the medicine for about a
year and a half and I was weaned off the Mellaril.
 I had another manic episode and this time was diagnosed with
schizophrenia. This time I took Risperdal, Lithium, and Mellaril. I was
slowly weaned off the Risperdal, experienced bizarre thoughts and six
months later was in the hospital again. Now, the diagnosis was schizoaffective bi-polar disorder.
 Nothing was happening like I thought it should and I invested things with
too much meaning. It felt like I couldn't predict anything, especially the
most mundane things, which were happening around me. I also had a
dark nightmarish feeling.
Next, I went in and out of the hospital three consecutive times within a
short period of time. I only felt normal for two days one week-end during
the second hospitalization.
The community behavioral health unit arranged for me to go to the State
Hospital for three months. I was discharged, but nothing changed.
 A few months later, while I was on vacation in another state, I even ended
up in a state hospital there when my actions became erratic. I had
stopped taking my oral medication before the trip. In an effort to solve this
problem, I received an injection of Haldol decanoate, was discharged after
a week, and resumed my partial program in my home state. Nothing made*

sense and I was paranoid. I thought I was being tested and kept the fact that I was in my own world to myself. People were there for the sole purpose of testing me. Everything seemed to be just a prop or an act. I was now nineteen years old.

At this juncture, I began attributing everything to spiritual forces. When I was scheduled for the next Haldol decanoate shot, something remarkable occurred. First I refused the shot, and almost simultaneously experienced a real sense of forgiveness from past sins. I knew there was a God and that meant that things were normal again!

I was able to work for temp services for awhile. Later, I landed a seasonal job as a banquet server, and then enrolled in community college. I struggled to appear normal; I blocked out my feelings and stayed as factual as I could. The old nightmarish feeling came and went and within a month I signed myself back into the hospital so I could get some medication to keep me stable and normal. I had to leave college, of course.

Now, I was in a partial program and felt more normal every day. This feeling was especially strong upon awaking each morning. Although I was still experiencing thought blocks and I usually made inaccurate predictions about everyday events and happenings, I hoped these feelings would leave with time.

I reached a point when I was taking Risperdal when the good feeling I had each morning left. I needed more and more medicine. Later I began taking Zoloft and felt like my mental awareness levels were increasing. The doctor then prescribed Paxil for obsessional thoughts.

I signed myself into the hospital again and when I came out, the outpatient doctor gave me Zyprexa. This gave me a more stable mental state, but I was still out of touch with my emotions and feelings. I had cloudy thoughts and my reactions did not match situations.

Eventually another doctor prescribed Clozaril which allowed me to work consistently for eighteen months. This was the longest employment I'd had since my problems started. I was still out of touch with reality, although I struggled to tell myself things were normal. I felt things would get better if I found the right medicine.

I met a doctor that took time to listen and he said my opposite feelings might never improve. He adjusted the Clozaril with some other meds and *had almost exhausted all possibilities when I began to consider trying natural methods of dealing with my problem.*

I had an old copy of a Canadian Schizophrenic Journal that featured an article on orthomolecular treatment that seemed like what I needed. My family and I were excited and bought the vitamins listed, but knew we needed to find a doctor who could tell us how much to use and in what combinations. We wrote to the Journal first and asked for a referral and they sent us a list of doctors who subscribed to their magazine. I began calling and writing them to try and find a doctor who could help me. Eventually, I remembered talking with a psychiatrist several years before who used medicine and vitamins and he had mentioned the Princeton Bio Center and explained the types of testing they provided. I dialed the old number I found and discovered that they no longer did testing or even had a treatment center in operation. There were no doctors there anymore. Now, I learned, they only dispense vitamins. I had been so close to finding my answer! Disappointment flooded me, but I asked the kind voice on the phone if she could recommend a doctor who knew how to help me to use orthomolecular treatment. She recommended Dr. Bonnie Camo and as I copied down her name and number I began to feel hopeful.

On my first visit I sensed I was finally on the right path and what Dr. Camo proposed was going to be able to address my problems.

My family and I had always felt I had too much or too little of some brain chemicals and when the balance became critical I took a turn for the worse and ended up in the hospital.

I took a homeopathic remedy there that day at Dr. Camo's and left with another to mix with water to take daily. I had a list of vitamins and supplements that I bought and began taking the next day. I also started to follow The Blood Type Diet. My emotions that had been frozen began to reappear within a week and I felt elated!

On my second visit three months later, I looked and felt alive again! My sallow skin tones turned pink and rosy, unwanted pounds had melted away, old layers of illness and confusion seemed to be dissolving, and I had hope that I had not had before, since my long journey began so many years ago.

In time, my level of functioning improved and I was now able to work a regular part time shift doing prep cooking in a restaurant. I eventually landed a lawn care job that demanded lots of physical exercise, which also helped me to look and feel better.

I have to admit that I had my share of ups and downs and sometimes overreacted when it came to trying to sort out my feelings, emotions, and physical responses to the various medications I took and doctors who prescribed them. My body seemed to require traditional [conventional - BC] medications even though I longed to be able to use only natural ones. It is true to say that for over seven years I had visited numerous doctors and had received a laundry list of ineffective pharmaceutical solutions.

 On the other hand I had one homeopathic visit, received minute amounts of natural substances, began to use vitamins and supplements, eliminated unhealthy foods, and saw improvement within days! Whatever imbalances that caused my erratic behavior were tamed by this skilled doctor's response to my symptoms.

For the last nine years I have continued to take vitamins and supplements along with traditional medications, have been able to work consistently and have even completed two years of technical college. I have my own apartment and feel grateful that I am able to live a normal life. I cannot imagine how my life would have been had I not been introduced to Dr. Camo and the natural treatment plan that she recommended.

PH's Story –pyroluria

If I had not found a system that involves first having someone that really cares to listen and observe, I would always have had a hard time getting help and learning what supporting myself is truly about. Someone that has blood sugar problems and difficulty focusing is going to have a difficult time getting to the point. There are other factors involved but solving this first set of problems of fundamental stability is crucial to anything else that follows. This kind of listening is the first and most important factor to inspire the patient to be involved, which must be the case. I believe this is the main difference between conventional medicine: The body and individual person is left in rather than out. The <u>body</u> heals; not the doctor. The next helpful find was to understand that Pyroluria is not a disease. I was not looking for something to kill and make go away or hide. This was about my unique engine and how to make my own octane to become *more productive and connected. Some of the most powerful changes <u>did</u> <u>not</u> include something to take but what to let go of. There were real reasons for my behavior. And I could take responsibility to make changes within a partnership of body and mind. As I slowed, I had to learn to listen outwardly but also learn a whole new perception of listening to the body speak. Pain is not always something that is unwanted. And with patience and this new form of knowledge, there can be a new found stability that is real and traceable. If I wanted to be healthy with good friendships, I needed to see that my own person was not one chronically without controls. No one could tell me this. But I needed guidance toward knowing that my ideas about what I saw and experienced were not silly or grandiose. There was real hope.*

Something that I feel I could not have found anywhere else with the same kind of connection to Orthomolecular Medicine was the choice you made of Lycopodium. First I had to stop coffee for at least a month. I do not drink a lot of coffee but just the initial idea and discipline needed carried over to other procedures. And the quality of new thinking that always happens when I take Lycopodium cannot be easily defined. This was a higher type of thinking that was again real and from within me: Insightful. I believe I wouldn't have had the same results if I hadn't found Lycopodium and the connection to Pyroluria you made. Can't say enough.
What I found from going to a Naturopathic doctor, that was also crucial, was the fact that I was creating alcohol in my system. This led to learning more about my digestive system and how retention enemas could be helpful. My first <u>direct</u> comparison to what I could achieve in clarity came from this kind of therapy. One moment I could be very cloudy and as things were flushed out I could witness an abrupt change. My fingers were instantly lighter and could move with more dexterity. My mood and thoughts would shift immediately to a familiar person that I knew from time to time. I used to say that "I get glimpses". Now I could see that my norm was based on toxic elements staying in my system too long. Those glimpses were actually the healthy perception I could achieve: In other words, the real me. Comparisons like this are very telling: Like standing in a busy street and the traffic goes away. No drama. What a novel idea!

This gave me more interest in learning to relax. If I could relax, I could let things go. I could think clearly and less confused more regularly. Diet became much more than just "eating healthy". And healthy became more than just not being sick. . Thank you for all your help.

Chapter 14

Autism and Mercury

Defeat Autism Now (DAN) is an organization of parents of autistic children, and physicians, (many of them also parents of autistic children), who believe that autism is curable, and have cured many children of this devastating disorder, through diet, nutrients, and detoxification. Autism was once an obscure disorder, supposed a half century ago to be caused by a cold, unfeeling, "refrigerator" mother. It now affects two percent of all children in the United States.

Minimata Disease

In the mid-1950's, in Minimata, Japan, a strange epidemic began. Symptoms started with peripheral sensory loss, muscle pain and tremors, difficulty speaking, and eventually loss of vision and hearing, leaving the victim cut off from the world, from which they soon departed. This new devastating disorder was found to be caused by high mercury levels in fish, a staple food of the area. Methyl mercury easily crosses the placenta, and infants were born severely mentally retarded, blind and deaf.   Minimata Bay had been polluted by mercury-laden industrial waste from a plastics company.   Minimata Disease, (mercury poisoning), is now widespread in third world countries like Brazil, where mercury is used for gold mining and other industries.

In "first world" country America, since 1990, the epidemic of autism is also leaving children unable to communicate, virtually deaf and blind to their surroundings and unable to recognize or communicate with other human beings. Again the culprit is thought by some to be mercury, given in well-meaning injections as a preservative (thimerosal) in vaccinations
to prevent childhood infections. (Thimerosal has now been removed from most immunizations, but is still present in some, like the flu vaccine.)

 Mercury from a mother's "silver" fillings can also pass through the placenta into the fetus. Pregnant women are also warned to limit their consumption of fish, (one of the most important sources of brain nutrients), due to its mercury content.

Although the mercury theory is denigrated by conventional medicine in favor of genetic explanations, it is impossible to have an epidemic of a genetic disorder. Evolution doesn't work that way. Although there is probably a genetic susceptibility, in the form of a decreased ability to remove heavy metals and other toxins, this was not a problem until heavy metals like mercury became so widespread in our environment.

Mercury in Your Teeth

In the 1820's silver amalgam (fifty percent mercury) was introduced by dentists to America as a cheaper substitute for gold in fillings. The dental community was polarized until 1899, when the pro-amalgam forces won out and formed the American Dental Association, which still endorses mercury amalgam "silver" fillings. Most people of my generation have gone through life with a mouthful of these. Many common diseases of aging like Alzheimer's, hormonal imbalances like hypothyroidism, autoimmune disorders, chronic fatigue, fibromyalgia, and psychological problems as listed below are now thought to be at least partly related to mercury and other toxic heavy metals.

Symptoms of mercury poisoning, as previously mentioned, include memory loss, shyness, timidity, loss of will power, indecision, lack of confidence, apathy and violent impulses. Autism may be considered an extreme expression of these tendencies, leaving the victim isolated in an "empty fortress", (a term used by Bruno Bettelheim, originator of the "refrigerator mother" theory.)

The DAN protocol for autism usually begins with diet free of wheat (gluten) and dairy (casein), as well as sugar. A mercury-poisoned body in its wisdom may encourage the growth of Candida yeast, which may incorporate some of the mercury into its cell walls. But Candida, which lives on sugar, leads to a "leaky gut" which allows absorption of undigested food particles, resulting in food allergies and digestive disorders. Many autistic children cannot properly digest gluten or casein, instead reducing these proteins to peptides that act like morphine in the brain. No wonder these children are not in touch with the world.

DAN doctors routinely test for mercury, lead, and other heavy metals in hair and urine. Diet, nutritional supplements, herbs, homeopathy, and sulfur-containing prescription medications like DMSA and DMPS can all be used to help remove mercury and other toxins from the body. The herb Cilantro, often used in Mexican food, also helps remove mercury. DAN no longer exists as an organization, but doctors trained in these methods and following the DAN protocol are still succeeding in restoring many autistic children to normal. High doses of injected methyl B_{12}, developed by Dr James Neubrander, have proven to be extremely successful.

The Homeopathic Cure

Homeopathic remedies, chosen to match the patient's constitution and symptoms, can enhance the body's healing powers and have cured some cases of autism, as described in <u>Impossible Cure</u> by Amy Lansky. On the other hand, a high level of mercury in the body is one of the "obstacles to cure" that can interfere with the action of homeopathic remedies.

Besides dental amalgams and mercury-based preservatives in vaccinations and other pharmaceuticals, the third major source of mercury in the environment is coal-burning power plants.

Fish – Good or Bad?

Eating low on the food chain is better for you and better for the planet. But omega-3 essential fatty acids, mostly found in fish and seafood, are vitally necessary for the brain and heart. Now we are told to limit fish to once a week, (or once a month if pregnant), due to its high mercury content.

If you eat fish, choose small fish like sardines, wild salmon and tilapia. Tuna and swordfish are large predator fish high in mercury that should be

94

eaten rarely if at all. One way to get the long chain EPA and DHA needed by the brain and heart is to buy fish oil capsules, purified to remove mercury and other toxins, at your health food store. Another good source is Krill oil, made from tiny shrimp low on the food chain, and very low in toxins.

Mercury Retrogression

"Mercury Retrograde", my astrological friends tell me, is when the planet Mercury appears to move backwards, relative to the other planets. At these times, communications may go awry. This may be a metaphor for real life mercury, the toxic heavy metal, which interferes with human communication and speech development, and causes retrogression of our higher mental functions.

Aluminum in Vaccines Causes Autism

It has recently been discovered that aluminum, which has been used for decades as an "adjuvant" in vaccines may be as bad or even worse than mercury. Autopsies on the brains of autistic people who died of various causes at various ages, done by Dr Christpher Exley, were all extremely high in aluminum, compared to brains of normal people. Aluminum, a known neurotoxin, is used in most vaccines as an adjuvant, to cause a stronger reaction. This is very strong evidence that this heavy metal is implicated in autism. The plausible mechanism has also been discovered. It was thought that the aluminum in vaccines remained at the injection site, but it is now known that it is taken up by macrophages which travel to the brain causing activation of microglia, inflammation and increased IL-6 cytokine levels, which impairs neurodevelopment and causes symptoms of autism. There are no studies showing the safety of aluminum adjuvants in vaccines, it was just assumed. An outrageous fraud by the pharmaceutical companies is the use of aluminum adjuvants in the placebos used in trials for FDA approval. They're comparing vaccines containing aluminum with placebos containing aluminum, so it looks like the vaccine is as safe as an inert placebo.

RM's Story: mercury poisoning
I first became aware of the Princeton Brain Bio Center about thirty

years ago. My aunt, Mary, who was my father's older sister, had some kind of condition for a number of years. She was frail, nervous, and had to wear a high neck brace for many years. She went to all the "best" doctors in New York and Boston (she lived in Wellesley Hills, Massachusetts) but nobody could figure out what was the problem. She was probably almost sixty years old then. One year we visited and I was amazed to see her strong and without her neck brace. I asked what happened and she told me about the PBBC. She had gone to see Dr. Pfeiffer and he had diagnosed her as suffering from a reaction to some trace metal. (Unfortunately, I don't know which one.) He was able to cure it with diet and vitamin therapy and without medication. The difference between before and after was almost unbelievable. Naturally, I was terribly impressed.

Her condition never recurred and she never wore a neck brace again. She was healthy until about age 84 or so when she was diagnosed with Alzheimer's. She died two years ago at about age 87.

My second PBBC story is about my mother. About twenty-five years ago, she became weak, she had digestive problems, and her palms and soles turned brown and wrinkled. Again, she went to all the "best" doctors in New York but to no avail. None of them had a clue. Knowing about my Aunt Mary's success, my mother went to see Dr. Pfeiffer and he diagnosed her as suffering from mercury poisoning. He treated her with vitamin therapy, had her reduce her intake of fish (she ate a lot of fish then, especially tuna and swordfish), and she had her amalgam fillings removed by a dentist in Denver, Colorado, who specialized in that. My mother was cured and her condition never recurred. Although she now has osteoporosis and has fallen and broken bones a number of times, she is still otherwise healthy at age 83 and living in New York.

Chapter 15

Heavy Metal Brain Damage

Lead poisoning is thought to have led to the downfall of the Roman Empire. The ancient Roman water pipes were made of up to 99.3% lead, according to Dr. K-G Wenzel in <u>The Earth's Gift to Medicine</u>. (I actually saw the remains of some of these lead pipes on a recent visit to Pompeii, the Roman city buried by the eruption of Vesuvius in 79 AD.) The upper classes also used lead-containing glazes on their ceramic drinking vessels. It seems probable that lead was a factor in the rise and fall of insane, murderous emperors like Nero and Caligula.

Serial Killers and Mass Murderers

In the Twentieth Century, Dr. William Walsh, former head of the Argonne National Laboratory near Chicago, found high lead levels in the hair analysis of all serial killers and mass murderers he tested. Serial killers would be classed as sociopaths, people who lack a conscience and empathy, and kill methodically and with premeditation. Mass murderers, on the other hand, seem normal until they suddenly snap under extreme stress, go insane and shoot everybody in a McDonald's, for instance. Dr. Walsh found both types high in cadmium as well as lead, and low in zinc. The mass murderers also tended to have high copper. Walsh later went on to found the Pfeiffer Treatment Center (PTC), named after my mentor, Dr. Carl Pfeiffer, with whom he collaborated. The PTC tests and treats people for heavy metals, vitamin and mineral deficiencies and other imbalances related to mental and physical illnesses.

Nature or Nurture?

Zinc deficiency is common in the general public in the US and in the Middle East. Dr. Pfeiffer speculated that this could be a factor in the warlike, violent nature of these areas. Dr. Walsh was on the Phil Donohue television show many years ago, and was asked which was more important in producing violent behavior, heredity or environment. He answered that it was a combination of a bad chemistry and a bad childhood.   It is interesting to note that the crime rate in the US went down sharply eighteen years after Roe versus Wade legalized abortion in 1973, according to <u>Freakonomics</u>, by Steven Levitt and Stephen Dubner. Apparently many women who want an abortion realize that they do not have the emotional or financial resources necessary to raise a healthy child, or they may not be able to be a good a mother to an unwanted child they were forced to give birth to.

Another explanation of why the crime rate went down in cities all over America in the 1990s was the removal of lead from gasoline starting in the 1970s. Lead is known to cause brain damage, especially in small children, who are low to the ground where lead from exhaust lurks and settles. Crime started going down in the '90s, when toddlers who were exposed to less lead had grown up and not become criminals. Each US state removed lead on its own schedule, and those who removed it sooner saw crime decrease sooner. Lead damages the parts of the brain that make us human - the pre-frontal cortex where we make executive decisions, the empathy circuits, areas that control aggression, etc. Kevin Drum at Mother Jones wrote the definitive argument for the lead/crime link. Today, leaded gasoline is banned in 175 countries, and there's been a decline in lead blood levels by about 90 percent.
The timing matches up: crime rose in the mid-to-late-20th century as cars spread around the world, and started to decline in the 70s as leaded gasoline was being outlawed.

Zinc vs Lead

Low zinc is associated with anger, hostility and verbal abuse, according to The Crazy Makers, by Carol Simontacchi, perhaps because low zinc allows lead and cadmium to rise. Many brain enzymes require zinc for activation. Dr. Pfeiffer studied lead-poisoned battery workers in the 1970's, and was able to bring their lead levels down to normal, using two grams of vitamin C and sixty milligrams of zinc daily for twenty-four weeks, even while they continued to work at the lead battery factory.

Low zinc in children can cause delayed puberty and short stature, since zinc is needed for production of testosterone, and for normal growth. Before subjecting a short child to expensive and uncomfortable growth hormone injections, zinc status should be assessed. A few cents worth of zinc daily could solve the growth problem, along with acne and poor immunity due to zinc deficiency.

Toxic Tobacco

One of the main sources of cadmium toxicity is tobacco smoking. Cadmium is thought to contribute to emphysema. Smoking also depletes vitamin C, which is needed to help prevent cancer and, along with zinc, to help excretion of heavy metals. Other sources of cadmium are refined foods, which have a low zinc to cadmium ratio, and old galvanized water pipes, made with zinc that was contaminated with cadmium. Newer water pipes made of copper seemed like a good substitute, but copper levels can go too high, especially with acidic well water. Greenish-blue stains in the sink and tub are a warning sign of high copper levels.

Copper, unlike lead and cadmium, is an essential mineral, but excessive amounts can lead to hypertension, depression, hyperactivity, headaches and other disorders. Many commercial multivitamins have too much copper. Chocolate is also quite high in copper. Two milligrams is considered the daily requirement, but this does not take into consideration the copper that is being absorbed from food and water.

Iron is another mineral that is essential, for formation of hemoglobin that carries oxygen to the brain and other organs, but can become toxic in excess. Men and postmenopausal women should make sure that their multivitamins are iron-free. Iron and copper are "oxidants", which promote aging, and act in opposition to antioxidant minerals like zinc and selenium.

Autistics on Opium?

Dr. Walsh describes a genetic disorder called metallothionein (MT) deficiency. MT requires zinc for activation, and helps bind and remove mercury, cadmium, and excess copper. MT binds to toxic metals in the intestinal lining and prevents their absorption. MT increases availability of zinc, which is needed to produce digestive enzymes that help break down casein and gluten, which otherwise are only partially digested to produce peptides called caseomorphine and gluteomorphine, which act like opium in the brain. These opioid peptides are thought to be one reason for the unresponsiveness of autistic people. This explains why many autistics do much better on a wheat and dairy free diet. MT also prevents intestinal yeast overgrowth and inflammation, which are common problems for people on the autistic spectrum.

Autism and other disorders affecting the brain, like attention deficit hyperactivity disorder (ADHD), obsessive compulsive disorder (OCD), bipolar disorder and schizophrenia, which seem to have a hereditary component, result from a bad combination of genetic abnormalities like MT deficiency, and the high levels of toxic heavy metals in the environment, which these people are unable to detoxify.

Iodine

Of course, heavy metals and other toxic elements also damage the rest of the body, not only the brain. Iodine used to be used in the flour-making process in the US. In the 1960's one slice of bread provided the recommended daily allowance (RDA) of 150 mcg of iodine. Then, about forty years ago, because of unfounded fears that people were getting too much iodine, it was replaced by bromine. Now most Americans probably suffer from bromine toxicity, as well as iodine deficiency.

In addition to bromine, Americans are also exposed to chlorine and fluoride in the water supply. These three elemental substances all belong to the chemical group called the halogens, to which iodine also belongs; therefore they antagonize iodine, which is needed to produce thyroid hormones. This may be one of the reasons for the epidemic of hypothyroidism and obesity in the US in the past three decades.

Iodine and Breast Cancer

Some researchers, such as Guy Abraham MD (best known for characterizing the different varieties of premenstrual syndrome and their treatments), believe that iodine deficiency is also a major contributing factor to the high rate of breast cancer in the US. Women in Japan who average 13.8 milligrams of iodine daily in their diet, which is rich in fish and seaweed, have a very low incidence of breast cancer. Even iodized salt in the US contains a miniscule amount of iodine, not enough to prevent hypothyroidism or breast cancer. And many people these days are avoiding salt altogether, or eating processed foods that are high in salt, but not the iodized variety.

The best dietary sources of iodine are seafood and seaweed (also known as sea vegetables) such as kelp, kombu, nori, arame, wakame, and dulse, which are all available at your local health food store. Dulse, sautéed in olive oil, tastes deliciously like bacon, but is much healthier.

Dr.Abraham's company, Optimox, has formulated a convenient supplement of iodine and iodide in optimum amounts and proportions, called Iodoral 12.5 mg. This is the same amount supplied by two drops of Lugol's solution, which has been used as an iodine supplement for over one hundred fifty years. An inexpensive test for determining iodine deficiency is described in a new book called <u>Iodine,</u> by Dr. David Brownstein, who has also written books on natural hormones, which are available on the internet, as is Iodoral.

The Iodine Test

The test is done by collecting urine for 24 hours after taking a dose of fifty milligrams of iodine, and measuring the amount of iodine excreted in the urine. People with sufficient iodine will excrete about 90 percent, or 45 mg of the ingested iodine. A person who is low in iodine will retain more of the load and their excretion rate will be less than 90 percent.

Dr. Brownstein has tested nearly five thousand patients for iodine levels, finding more than 96 percent to be low or severely deficient. He considers iodine deficiency an epidemic in the United States, with consequences such as lowered intelligence, attention deficit hyperactivity disorder (ADHD), infertility, thyroid disorders, and cancer of the breast, thyroid and reproductive organs.

Chapter 16

Natural Help for Arthritis

Arthritis in its various manifestations affects up to fifty-five million Americans. The most common form is osteoarthritis, also called degenerative joint disease, which rarely begins before age forty, but eventually affects fifty to eighty-five percent of people over sixty-five. "Wear and tear" is part of the picture, since it often begins where there has been an injury or trauma earlier in life.   Osteoarthritis is a progressive degeneration of cartilage, the smooth, slippery substance covering the ends of bones; it degenerates faster than the body can regenerate it. Each joint in your body is encased in a capsule covered by a membrane. The membrane secretes synovial fluid to lubricate the joint. Too little fluid causes stiffness, while too much causes swelling.

Arthritis affects nearly everyone, if they live long enough. It is not a new disorder. Anthropologists have found indications of osteoarthritis in the fossil bones of the original caveman, the Neanderthals, and even in dinosaur bones. Medical science has not yet discovered the cause, or even a good treatment. Three times as many women as men are affected. The weight-bearing joints -- knees, hips and back -- and the hands are most affected. The muscles, the tendons attaching muscles to bones, and the ligaments that attach bone to bone, all lose strength and elasticity, and joints become stiff and painful. Even bones are affected, becoming brittle and easier to break. Unlike the more severe and less common rheumatoid arthritis, which affects younger people, there are no laboratory tests for common (osteo) arthritis. The onset is gradual. There is intermittent pain on motion of the affected joints, often aggravated by weather, diet, overuse, and stress.

Conventional treatment usually involves aspirin or aspirin-like drugs called non-steroidal anti-inflammatory drugs (NSAIDs), and/or steroid drugs, to relieve inflammation and pain. But these drugs may cause more harm than good. NSAIDs interfere with the joints' ability to produce proteins needed to build cartilage, and destroy enzymes needed to manufacture chondroitin, a major component of cartilage. Arthritic joints absorb more NSAIDs than normal joints, causing even more damage, in a vicious cycle of degeneration and pain. NSAIDs also damage the stomach lining and can lead to ulcers. Steroid drugs like prednisone are even worse, causing a five-fold increase in death of cells that make chondroitin. They also suppress the immune system, producing increased susceptibility to infection, and accelerate osteoporosis.

Herbal Treatments

Many herbs are available that have anti-inflammatory effects that can ease joint symptoms without the side effects of conventional drugs. Ashwaganda, boswellia, cat's claw, feverfew, ginger, and willow bark are popular choices. (Do not take cat's claw if you are on insulin for diabetes.) Cayenne pepper in the form of capsaicin cream applied to the affected areas causes brief skin pain that counteracts chronic pain. Clematis raises the pain threshold. Kava kava, an herb from the South Pacific, relieves pain and helps promote restful sleep. Turmeric is the primary anti-inflammatory herb of Ayurvedic medicine. Curcumin is its main chemical component, which relieves pain and inflammation and scavenges free radicals.

Moderate exercise is beneficial to strengthen bones and increase muscle mass to help support the joints, and to help control excess weight which puts more stress on joints. Swimming or exercising in warm water is an excellent way to keep joints mobile without putting stress on them. Many community pools have "aquacise" programs that benefit arthritis sufferers.

Homeopathy

Homeopathic medicine is a gentle and highly effective form of treatment that helps the body heal itself. Discovered two hundred years ago by German physician Samuel Hahnemann, it is based on the principle of "like cures like", or the "Law of Similars", which states that the best medicine for any set of symptoms in a sick person is the substance that would produce the same set of symptoms if given to a healthy person.

One of the homeopathic remedies most commonly used for arthritis is *Rhus toxicodendron*, for pain with stiffness that is worse when first beginning to move, and improves with continued movement. The pain is relieved by warmth, and aggravated by cold, wet weather. Another remedy is *Bryonia*, for swollen joints with sharp pain that is aggravated by the slightest movement. The patient is irritable and angry if touched or disturbed. The pain is relieved by pressure, so they prefer to lie on the painful side. They have a dry mouth and are very thirsty.

Arnica montana is the first remedy to take for any injury or physical trauma. It is useful for a sore, bruised feeling in the joints or muscles, for overexertion, and even for jet lag. *Rhododendron* is for musculoskeletal pain that wanders from joint to joint, and is much worse before and during a storm. *Causticum*, on the other hand, is good for arthritic symptoms that actually improve in wet, rainy weather and are worse on cold, dry windy days. It is useful for contracted, shortened tendons and joint deformity. The patient who needs this remedy tends to be an idealistic rebel against authority.

"Deadly" Nightshades

Your diet may affect progression of arthritis. Many people are sensitive to so-called "nightshade" vegetables: potatoes, tomatoes, eggplants and peppers, (which are in the same botanical family as deadly nightshade.)

They contain a toxin called solanine. It may take up to three months of avoidance to know whether nightshades affect you.   According to Dr. Norman Childers, of Rutgers University, who discovered this effect of nightshades in the 1970's, about seventy percent of arthritis sufferers found relief on a nightshade free diet.

Another consideration is the amount and type of fat in the diet. Meat from land animals (beef, pork, and lamb) is high in saturated fat which causes inflammation in the body. On the other hand, fish, especially from cold northern waters, contains anti-inflammatory omega-3 unsaturated fat. Salmon and sardines are excellent choices. Wild salmon is preferable to farm-raised, but it is expensive and hard to find. Fortunately, canned salmon is all wild-caught, and much cheaper than fresh. It can be substituted for tuna to make a healthier fish salad. Tuna, like other large, predatory fish, is high in mercury and should be used sparingly. Organic eggs, especially from chickens allowed to run free and eat wild plants and insects, which increases their omega-3 and vitamin content, are also good to include in the diet.

Sulfur Supplements

Supplements that supply building blocks for cartilage may be helpful. Glucosamine sulfate and chondroitin sulfate are very popular, and many people find them effective. Methylsulfonylmethane (MSM) also helps build cartilage, as well as synovial fluid, and decreases inflammation.   Two thousand milligrams per day is a reasonable amount. MSM is a derivative of dimethylsulfoxide (DMSO), which is used externally, to quench free radicals and increase effectiveness of the body's cortisol. DMSO often gives immediate pain relief. The only side effect is making you smell like garlic.

S-adenosyl methionine (SAMe) is an activated form of the amino acid methionine, first used in Italy over thirty years ago. It is useful for arthritis and fibromyalgia, as well as depression. It is rather expensive, but effective. Start with 400 mg twice a day for at least three weeks, and then reduce to 200 mg twice a day for maintenance.

Vitamin B3, in the form of niacinamide, was found by Dr. William Kaufman in the 1940's to help relieve arthritic pain. He found it worked best in small frequent doses, 250 mg every three hours, six times a day. The other form of B3, niacin, also works. It produces a "flush", warmth and redness of the skin, by dilating the blood vessels and increasing circulation, which is thought to help remove toxins from the body. The flush, which could be scary if you were not expecting it, is normal and harmless, only lasts 20 minutes, and is enjoyed by many.

Other useful anti-inflammatory supplements include vitamin C, 1000 milligrams two or three times a day, vitamin E 400 international units (iu) per day, and vitamin A 10,000 iu or beta carotene 15mg. Important minerals include zinc 30 to 50 mg daily, manganese 30 mg daily (less if blood pressure is high), and selenium 200 mcg daily.   Copper 2 mg daily may be needed (unless your copper level is high.) Vitamin D has recently been found to be needed in much greater amounts than previously thought. At least 1000 iu per day may help prevent osteoarthritis, as well as osteoporosis. Vitamin K_2 works with vitamin D_3 to prevent osteoporosis and coronary artery disease by keeping calcium in the bones and out of the arteries. Unlike vitamin K_1, which is found in green vegetables, K_2 occurs in animal products like eggs, cheese and meat, especially grass-fed.

Chapter 17

Prevent Breast Cancer with Ayurveda

I highly recommend a wonderful book called <u>Waking the Warrior Goddess</u> by Christine Horner MD, about preventing and fighting breast cancer using the principles of Ayurveda, an ancient healing system from India. *Ayur* means life and *veda* means knowledge. Ayurveda means "the knowledge of life." This holistic system of medicine, at least five thousand years old, is based on maintaining balance in your physiology. It is the source of many techniques used in alternative medicine today, such as yoga, massage, meditation, herbs, breathing, diet and detoxification. Dr. Horner uses the metaphor of the Warrior Goddess for the body's innate healing capacity.

"Food is medicine" was a basic Ayurvedic principle thousands of years before Hippocrates said it. Fruits and vegetables are "virtual anticancer pharmacies." Phytochemicals in plants have many ways of protecting you from cancer. Carotenoids which give color to red, orange and yellow fruits and vegetables are potent antioxidants and block different steps in development of cancer. All cruciferous vegetables, like broccoli, cabbage and kale, contain indole-3 carbinole, which stops breast cancer cells from growing, and converts estrogen into a non-cancer-promoting form. Broccoli also contains sulforaphane, which promotes liver enzymes which destroy carcinogens and move them out of the body. Of course, all these fruits and vegetables should be organic, so you are not introducing more carcinogenic pesticides into your body.

Whole grains are rich in vitamins, minerals, fiber and lignans, all of which are protective against cancer, as well as heart disease and diabetes. Research shows that eating a high fiber diet decreases the risk of breast cancer by half. Flax seeds are the richest plant source ofomega-3 fatty acids, which lower cancer risk by damping inflammation which initiates cancer, heart disease and arthritis. Flax seeds have one hundred times more lignans than any other food. Lignans make the breast more resistant to toxins, prevent cancer cells from growing, and help prevent metastasis. Lignans also decrease production of forms of estrogen which promote cancer, and increase beneficial forms of estrogen.

Green tea is the number one anticancer beverage, full of anti-inflammatories and antioxidants, such as polyphenols like ECGC. A powerful anticancer spice is turmeric, the brilliant yellow-orange root used in curries and in Ayurvedic and Chinese medicine for over five thousand years. Turmeric destroys toxins in the liver, is powerfully anti-inflammatory and antioxidant, and prevents DNA mutations that lead to cancer. Turmeric also helps expel gallstones, improves digestion, lowers cholesterol and plaque, and promotes wound healing. Its main active ingredient is curcumin, which is available in capsules. It works best if taken along with whole turmeric.

What about Meat?

Eating red meat may be a serious risk factor for breast cancer. When animal protein is cooked, especially at high heat, like frying, carcinogens are formed. Saturated animal fat is converted into a carcinogen by bacteria in your large intestine. Animal fat is also the storage site for all the pesticides on the food the animal ate, as well as the antibiotics, hormones, and growth stimulants the animals were given. Grilling meat adds additional carcinogens. Sugar is cancer cells' favorite food. Stevia is a safe substitute for sweetening.

Sleep Heals

Ayurveda teaches that proper sleep is essential to good health. During sleep the mind/body is repaired and purified. In darkness the pineal gland produces melatonin, which promotes natural sleep and is a powerful cancer preventer. The best melatonin production occurs when you go to bed by 10 pm and get up by 6 am.

Exercise lowers your risk of breast cancer, in part by helping prevent obesity which increases your risk. Aerobic exercise causes the brain to produce healing neuropeptides which reduce stress and prevent depression. Yoga, an ancient part of Ayurveda, facilitates the union of your mind/body and breath. Yoga reduces anxiety, fatigue, tension and stress, and promotes mental function. Yoga reduces the stress hormone cortisol, and promotes the alpha brainwave state, where the left and right hemispheres work together. Yoga is a form of meditation. Other forms of meditation, such as transcendental meditation, promote health, balance, and "negate old age and disease."For more information, read the book, or go to www.drchristinehorner.com for a free video or DVD with important lifesaving techniques for preventing breast cancer.

JS's Story – breast cancer

I never seriously believed I would develop cancer. During those early days, most of the diagnostic process seemed surreal to me. Even as I viewed the sonogram and saw the gray spot with white lines stretching from it, staring from the screen at me, or entered a darkened office to view a line of my backlight mammogram films, I struggled to claim this disease as my own. A week later a needle biopsy confirmed that the lump in my left breast was indeed malignant. Despite last year's film being clear, now I looked intently at a dark mass that measured two centimeters. No one in my family had ever been diagnosed with cancer and I had zero risk factors, personally. What would I do?
Later, I received the standard treatment options at my first appointment with a surgeon. Fresh from that appointment, with those verbal remarks echoing in my ears, I headed for an appointment with Dr. Camo. I had initially made this homeopathic appointment because of menopausal symptoms, but when the cancer diagnosis surfaced, that took center stage. The timing was perfect and what first appeared to be a conflict,

actually turned into a blessing. After hearing the surgeon's plans and prognosis, it was so beneficial to actually receive the natural counterpart of his view. Now, I heard a vastly different approach that offered to build up my immune system, help my body to heal itself, and to improve my over-all heath, all while using harmless, natural substances. Homeopathy offered the opportunity to hope and not to fear. Dr. Camo explained Dr. Ramakrishnan's plusing method of using two homeopathic remedies alternately. One, carcinosin, was made from a breast cancer cell, and the second, sepia, was termed my constitutional remedy. I began the first two-and- a-half hour process the following day. In addition, I started a cancer prevention diet which consisted of eating fresh, organic vegetables, meat, and eggs, adding specific foods known to be good for treating cancer, while avoiding processed foods and empty calorie items. I also eliminated coffee and soft drinks from my diet and basically drank only green, black or herbal teas and spring water. Another strategy I embraced was drinking Essiac Tea, which is known for its cancer fighting properties. I learned how to brew the tea and conscientiously drank it three times daily. The vitamins and supplements that Dr. Camo prescribed helped to make my body inhospitable to cancer and gave me another weapon in my battle.

During this time I read many books and articles on natural medicine and I learned about various methods others used to help their bodies fight the disease and recover their health.

While undergoing preadmission testing at my local hospital, about one week after I began my homeopathic regimen, I experienced shooting pain and a scratching sensation at the tumor site. I learned this was my immune system attacking the tumor. I felt empowered and hopeful, sensing this was a positive occurrence.

I did have a lumpectomy two weeks after my diagnosis and then due to an unclear margin, had another surgery in another four weeks to remove more suspicious cells. After the surgery I experienced a tremendous energy surge. Maybe since the tumor was gone my body now had energy to spare.

Two diagnostic procedures I learned about in Cancer Diagnosis, by W. John Diamond, M.D. and W. Lee Cowden, M.D, the Therma-Scan and the Anti Malignant Antibody Screen (AMAS) helped me to gauge my own health over a longer time period. The Therma-Scan uses infrared photography to show areas emitting excessive heat, which may signal malignant disease. I began these tests within a year after my surgeries. The first showed a large area of vascular tissue that had been formed to support the tumor. Dr. Camo increased the potency of my homeopathic remedies and after taking the new dose for three months the second

Therma-Scan showed a noticeable reduction in the size and extent of the area. Again I could actually feel the area constrict and pulse while I was taking the remedies.

The AMAS is a special type of blood test that checks for specific antibodies formed against cancer. By noting the presence or absence of antibodies, one can compare normal or abnormal ranges of the antibodies and thus assess the situation. My results were always within the normal range that signaled no sign of cancer.

In an effort to prevent further cancer risks I began eliminating cancer-causing chemicals not only from my diet, but also from my environment. I only bought food, make-up, shampoos, toothpaste and cleaning products that were strictly natural and/or organic. In order to avoid exposure to harsh chemicals, I even took my own shampoo and conditioner to my hair stylist. I continued taking my remedies daily for over three years and have never stopped taking the vitamins, supplements, and drinking Essiac Tea at least once a day.

In addition to remedies and vitamins, three intangible assets helped me a great deal; Faith, Hope, and Humor.

My personal faith grew, during those days of uncertainty. I felt I was not alone in making decisions and understanding my options, and ultimately recognized that I may indeed succumb to cancer. Complete healing was completely possible, too! One morning before my husband left for work we read a devotional that included the Bible verse Jeremiah 29:11, "I know the plans that I have for you, declares the Lord…, plans to give you a hope and a future…" I was overwhelmed by how appropriate this message was for me and my family at that moment. I grasped these words as assurance that I would indeed live and be able to set goals for that promised future.

Hope is another very real antidote that I discovered during this battle.

The head start I gained from homeopathic remedies, supplements, and organic food helped me to maintain a positive attitude. I began exercising right after my surgery, didn't miss a day of teaching, and found comfort in looking ahead to the future. I actually seemed to gain strength and vitality from watching my young students work. During this time I completed a research project that I had been avoiding and then enrolled in graduate school. I knew having a goal would be good medicine for me, as well. I spent the next three years earning my Masters degree in Education.

Humor was also a very powerful tool in my fight to recover my health. Once, before I had conclusive information, I was feeling overwhelmed by the uncertainties of my case when I began watching the movie Mrs. Doubtfire. I started laughing at Robin Willams' antics and felt the bad feelings, fear, and anxiety, just lift from my spirit. My surprised husband, who just minutes before was trying to console me, heard my laughter, stopped what he was doing and gratefully joined me.

Even though I didn't realize it at the time, my wellness plan had actually been set in motion several years before my diagnosis.
I joined an organic food co-op about three years before and as a result had been learning better, more natural ways of living. I used only stainless steel cookware, had a water filter installed on my kitchen faucet and had been following the Blood Type Diet. All of these separate steps greatly simplified the overall process of adopting a natural approach to wellness.

I refused to take radiation or chemo-therapy, even though both treatments were presented to me as the traditional, "next steps."
It was also comforting to realize that my body knew exactly where to send "killer cells" and was not dependent on a tattoo to guide a beam of radiation.
I'm sure those practitioners I saw were puzzled when I refused to sign up for further treatments from them, but I grew more confident from my own experience that I was indeed following the best treatment plan. Instead of being burned or poisoned, I was enjoying the best health I'd ever experienced as an adult! My skin glowed, my weight dropped to a healthy level without any extra measures and I had more energy than ever before. I know I laughed louder and longer and much more frequently during those days. I was able to relax and enjoy simple pleasures like trying new recipes, hiking in the woods, fishing, and letting my hair grow long, without feeling guilty. People often commented that I looked so much younger.

I'm truly thankful that Dr. Camo was there to guide me through the maze of conflicting advice I received and to help me learn the basics of making safe, healthy, effective choices. I truly believe that homeopathy provided me with the best possible solution. My positive experience has caused me to respond to any illness or discomfort by noting my symptoms and seeking a compatible homeopathic remedy. The body's symptoms provide clues to treat, as well as diagnose, its illnesses. Through homeopathy I took an active part in regaining my health and am positive I made the best decision I could have made.

Chapter 18

Flu Alternatives

Fall is flu time. Every year these stealth invaders make their way around the world, powered by coughs, sneezes, and handshakes, entering your body through mucous membranes in the eyes, nose and mouth. Within one to three days, the battle in your body results in fever, chills, weakness, aching muscles or joints, sore throat, cough, headache and loss of appetite. There may be a fever of 101 degrees or up to 104 which may last four or five days. Some flus also involve abdominal pain and diarrhea.

You are most contagious one day before symptoms start and up to seven days after. Complications are most common in infants, the elderly, and those with a compromised immune system. Each year, we are told, 36,000 people die in the US from the common seasonal flu and its complications. Flu subtypes are constantly changing. The vaccine is made every year from different subtypes based on what was prevalent in different parts of the world the year before. Recent studies have shown that the flu vaccine affords less than thirty percent protection in the elderly population which is most at risk for complications. In 2009, there was great fear that the new H1N1 "swine flu" would produce a severe epidemic, affecting mostly children, teenagers and young adults, unlike the usual seasonal flu. The fearful hype was overblown.

Many times when we feel like we have the flu, we actually have a flu-like illness caused by other viruses like Parainfluenza and Picornavirus.

Medical experts estimate that only fifteen percent of flu-like illness is actually caused by the flu virus. The other eighty-five percent, caused by those other viruses, are not prevented by the flu shot. Also, the flu vaccine is one of those which still contain the mercury preservative thimerosal, which has been linked with autism. Fortunately homeopathic remedies, nutrition, and healthy lifestyle can help prevent and relieve all types of colds and flu-like illnesses.

The first step in preventing colds and flus is a healthy diet and lifestyle. Wash your hands frequently and avoid touching your eyes and mouth. Stay away from sick people and crowded areas. Avoid stress or practice stress reduction techniques.

Exercise regularly and eat a diet high in vitamins and phytonutrients. We need all the colorful antioxidants found in fruits and vegetables. These are of course much more abundant and fresh in the summer, when no one gets the flu.

The immune system benefits from supplements like vitamin A, the carotenes, C, D, and zinc, found in a daily multivitamin. Most people can use vitamin C, 500 to 1000 mg twice a day, or every hour during acute infections. Zinc may be used in the form of lozenges of 10 to 15 mg taken every two hours at the first sign of a cold or flu, for a direct anti-viral effect. For daily use, do not exceed 30 mg per day unless advised by a health professional. Zinc is best taken with food to avoid possible nausea.

If you are hit by a cold or flu-like illness, use common sense. Get plenty of rest, drink lots of fluids, water, fresh juices, herbal teas, hot soups and broths. Extract or tea of Echinacea, the Purple Coneflower, first used by Native American Indians, is still one of the best immune enhancers. Elderberry has antiviral properties and reduces flu symptoms. Recent studies from Norway using Sambucol, an extract of Black Elderberry, confirm its benefits for flu symptoms.

Pizza Power?

Oregano oil has long been used in botanical medicine for prevention and treatment of infections, especially colds and respiratory infections. Recent studies show that oregano oil alone (Oreganol) or in combination with cumin, sage and cinnamon (Oregacillin) can markedly reduce the virulence of human influenza virus A2. These two products can also completely block replication of human coronavirus, the pathogen associated with Severe Acute Respiratory Syndrome (SARS). (<u>Holistic Primary Care</u>, Fall, 2004.)

A Healthy Brew

Even ordinary black tea kills viruses! Tea is loaded with antioxidants. Immunologists at Harvard University discovered that people who drank five cups of black tea a day for two weeks pumped up their immune system T-cells to produce ten times more interferon that fights cold and flu viruses. Green tea should also work.

There may be some truth to the old "Jewish penicillin" remedy, chicken soup, especially if made with lots of carotene-rich carrots, parsley full of vitamin A and C, and garlic, loaded with virus-fighting sulfur compounds. Laboratory research suggests that homemade and canned chicken soup contain anti-inflammatory substances that decrease symptoms like runny noses and coughs.

The best known homeopathic remedy for cold and flu symptoms is *Oscillococcinum*, made from the liver and heart of a duck. Ducks and other wild birds in places like China are thought to be reservoirs of all flu viruses that affect humans. Viruses can sometimes spread from ducks to chickens, and then to humans, causing the notorious "avian" or "bird flu", H5N1, that still threatens the world, in spite of thousands of chickens being killed in Asia to prevent its spread.

According to ABC TV news, reported on October 7, 2005, DNA studies on tissue preserved from 1918 flu victims indicate that it was caused by a bird flu virus. Since *Oscillo* contains all the viruses found in ducks, it should be a good choice for bird flu, as well as regular flu. *Oscillococcinum*, made by Boiron, is FDA approved and available in health food stores and pharmacies. It usually works if taken within 48 hours of the onset of symptoms. Clinical trials show that, if taken early on, it can relieve flu symptoms, including fever, chills and body aches, within 48 hours. It can also be used preventively once a month, or when you may have been exposed to someone with a cold or flu. It should also work for swine flu.

Another homeopathic preventive remedy is *Influenzinum*. Homeopathic pharmacies make it fresh each year from that year's flu vaccine. Studies conducted in India and England between 1968 and 1970 found it highly effective at preventing the flu. It may be taken once a month during the flu season. Studies suggest that it increases levels of immunoglobulins IgA and IgG, which help the body fight infections

There have been three serious worldwide flu epidemics in the Twentieth Century. The worst was the 1918 Spanish influenza epidemic that killed twenty-two million people worldwide. Five-hundred-thousand people died in the United States. Weakened populations due to stress and malnutrition in the wake of World War I may have been a factor in the ease and extent of its spread.   In the US only twenty percent of those treated by conventional medicine survived, while eighty percent of those treated by homeopathy survived. (<u>Homeopathy the Home Handbook for Survival</u>, Alan Schmukler, 2003)

Heavy use of aspirin newly patented by Bayer may have also been a factor in the high death rate. Many victims with blood-filled lungs, not a usual symptom of flu, could have been due to the anticoagulant effect of aspirin. Even the fever-lowering effect would have made it harder for the body to fight off the virus. Homeopaths did not prescribe aspirin.

Part 3

Homeopathic Medicine

Chapter 19

What is Homeopathy?

What is homeopathy? Homeopathy is a medical science that uses natural substances to simulate illness and stimulate healing. It is based on the principle that *like cures like.* Any substance that can produce symptoms in a healthy person can cure the same symptoms in a sick person.

Symptoms represent the body's best effort to heal itself. When you have a cold, your eyes and nose run because they are secreting more tears and mucus to wash out dead germs and white blood cells and the debris of the battlefield. Taking cold medicines to dry up secretions makes it more difficult for your body to fight the disease. The body's coughing and sneezing reflexes are also designed to expel pathogens from the respiratory tract. Cough suppressants interfere with this self-protective mechanism.

 A homeopathic way of treating a cold would be to take something that produces the same effect your body is exhibiting, like eating raw onions or garlic, as in the old Italian folk remedy. The tearing eyes and running nose caused by raw onions closely resemble the symptoms of a cold. It would certainly be more pleasant to take your raw onion in homeopathic form, as *Allium cepa*, one of the most commonly used remedies for colds, as well as allergies and hay fever with similar symptoms.

The Wisdom of the Body

The word homeopathy is derived from two Greek words: *homoios* which means similar, and *pathos* which means disease or suffering. Homeopathy treats disease with a substance that can *cause* the same or

similar symptoms. This at first may seem to make no sense. We are used to the conventional approach where every symptom is suppressed by a drug that causes the opposite effect. But symptoms are not merely derangements proving the body's stupidity, but rather an attempt at healing.

In infectious diseases, a fever is the body's deliberate resetting of its thermostat at a higher level to speed up the work of the immune system in fighting invading microbes. Taking a drug to lower a fever interferes with the body's self healing. (Of course, if a fever reaches dangerously high levels, it must be brought down, which can be accomplished quickly and safely with homeopathy.)

Homeopathy and Computers

Homeopathy has no side effects, but when the remedy is given, you may feel worse before you feel better. Homeopathic remedies cure by presenting the body with an energy pattern which mimics the energy pattern of the disease. This triggers exactly the correct healing response. Homeopathic remedies are made from natural substances, including poisonous substances, that are so highly diluted that they contain no actual molecules of the substance, only its energy pattern, or information. The remedy gives your body instructions for healing, analogous to the way a compact disc instructs a computer's hard drive.

Homeopathy has been made a lot easier by computers. The first homeopathic software program, called MacRepertory, was just starting to be developed when I started studying at the National Center for Homeopathy Summer School in 1995. We learned to "repertorize" the old fashioned way, looking up every symptom in a large book called a repertory, which lists thousands of symptoms and the remedies that have relieved them, organized by body parts and systems, that have been collected over the last two hundred years.

It used to take hours to do what a computer can now do in seconds. Of course, you can't automatically prescribe the first remedy the computer comes up with. It gives you possibilities to consider, which you then look up in the second of homeopathy's basic tools, another big book called a Materia Medica, which lists the most important of the three thousand or so remedies that have been proven so far.

"Proving" is a process developed by Samuel Hahnemann, the father of homeopathy, to discover what disorders a remedy can cure. He did the first proving on himself. He knew that Peruvian bark was one of the few medicines of his day that actually worked. It was a treatment for malaria, also known as intermittent fever. Peruvian bark, or cinchona, is the source of quinine, which is still used today as a treatment for malaria. Textbooks of the day (two hundred years ago) said it worked because of its bitter taste, but that made no sense to Hahnemann. Lots of things taste bitter and don't cure malaria. He started taking a dose of this South American wonder drug every day, and soon developed symptoms resembling malaria, which went away when he stopped taking it.

The Law of Similars

He had discovered a new principle of medicine, the ability of a substance that produces symptoms, to relieve similar symptoms in a sick person. He called this the Law of Similars. This idea can also be expressed in computer terminology as your condition being "highlighted", (by taking a substance that produces the same symptoms) and then "deleted". I also like to think of homeopathic remedies as working by "rebooting your human biocomputer." All the symptoms (mistakes) that have crept in, perhaps over a lifetime, can be removed by taking the correct remedy, returning your body to its previous functioning condition, a more perfect version of you, whatever your constitutional type is.

Homeopathic Potencies

Homeopathic remedies are available in various strengths known as potencies, made by diluting and succussing (shaking vigorously) or triturating (grinding with a mortar and pestle) the original substance. Hahnemann first began diluting remedies to reduce the toxicity and side effects of the herbs, minerals and poisons commonly used as medicine in his day. He discovered that the more he diluted a remedy, as long as it was succussed, the stronger and yet more gentle it became. A potency that is made by dissolving one part of the remedy in nine parts of water (or a water/alcohol mixture) is a one in ten dilution, called a 1X potency , from the Roman numeral for ten. When one part of this is combined with nine parts of water it becomes the 2X potency. This procedure can be continued indefinitely, always succussing between dilutions. After about 12 dilutions, it is likely that there are no actual molecules of the substance remaining; however, the energy of the original material remains in the water.

The C potencies (Roman numeral for one hundred), are made in a similar way, by serial dilution of one part to ninety-nine. Commonly used C strengths are 12C, 30C, 200C and 1000C (better known as 1M – the Roman numeral for one thousand). The higher potencies are used for mental symptoms and constitutional prescribing. Lower ones are used for more acute situations. If the potency is too high, it may produce an "aggravation", in which the symptoms become worse before they become better. This is often considered a good sign, proof that the remedy is working.

LM Potencies

Hahnemann's goal was always to cure without aggravation, to not make the patient suffer. In the sixth and final edition of his <u>Organon of Medicine,</u> completed just before his death in 1843, at the age of 89, he described a new method of making and taking remedies, which made everything else obsolete. He used a much higher dilution, one part in fifty thousand, known by the Roman numerals LM, with much less succussing, which

produced a much more effective, yet gentler cure. Due to various circumstances, the sixth edition was not published until 1920, and most homeopaths have never heard of it, and are still practicing according to the old methods. I was fortunate to learn about LM potencies early in my homeopathic career, from Dr. Luc DeSchepper, who was then teaching courses in New Jersey.   I used LM's with most of my patients and had very good results.

Chapter 20

Homeopathy for Children's Illnesses

Now that cough and cold medicines for young children have been taken off the market, where are parents to turn to help their little ones through these winter miseries? Of course, it was found that these drugs didn't work anyway; they just helped parents feel better while their child's immune system was fighting off the germs. These pharmaceuticals may even have interfered with the healing process, keeping the child ill longer. Many children these days are prone to recurrent ear infections, and have had multiple courses of antibiotics, which do little more than make germs stronger and kids weaker (and drug companies richer.) Antibiotics kill good normal intestinal bacteria along with the harmful ones, paving the way for candidiasis, leaky gut and food allergies. Many germs have become resistant to most or all antibiotics. Microbes evolve faster than new drugs can be developed. Homeopathy strengthens the immune system and can prevent the need for antibiotics. Germs can never develop a resistance to homeopathic remedies, because homeopathy works not by killing germs, but by stimulating the healing power of the body and the immune system. So of course, homeopathy also works on viruses, on which antibiotics have no effect.

Got Milk?

I find that many children are relieved of the tendency to frequent colds and ear infections by having all dairy products removed from their diets, even if milk, ice cream, yogurt or cheese (including pizza) are their favorite foods. Milk sensitivity is more common in people with Type O blood. This is not the same as lactose intolerance, and lactaid milk or tablets will not help. After a few months, some people may be able to reintroduce milk products, especially if they have had a homeopathic constitutional remedy to help normalize the immune system.

Homeopathy can be used for children's acute problems like earaches, sore throats, upset stomach, colic, fevers, teething, and injuries. It also works on behavior problems, learning problems, emotional trauma, fears, depression and anxiety. You don't even need to have a diagnosis. The choice of remedy is not based on the name of the illness, but on the symptoms. Symptoms are the body's way of telling you what it needs.

Remedy Clues

Changes in personality and behavior during illness are an important clue. Whatever the illness, if the child becomes weepy, clingy, complains of feeling hot, but is not thirsty, she will probably respond to *Pulsatilla*. If he is angry, irritable, impatient, and chilly, *Nux vomica* should work. If the child is anxious, restless, chilly, weak from any exertion, thirsty for small frequent sips, and worse between midnight and 3 am, *Arsenicum* is the remedy, whether the ailment is asthma, food poisoning or panic attacks.

Pulsatilla is a remedy for colds with thick, non-irritating, yellow or greenish mucus. The nose is more congested at night and lying down, and in a warm room. The mouth is dry, but the child is not thirsty. She becomes weepy and clings to her mother.

Aconitum is useful during the first 24 hours of a cold that starts suddenly after exposure to cold and wind. The child may wake after midnight with a dry, croupy cough, shortness of breath, and a mouth so dry he can't spit. The cough is worse from being cold or drinking cold water.

Belladonna should be in every parent's homeopathic emergency kit, for a high fever that develops suddenly in the middle of the night, with a hot head that radiates heat, while the hands and feet may be cold. The child's face, lips, tongue and ears are flushed red. The mouth and throat are dry,

but she is usually not thirsty. There may be a throbbing headache that comes on quickly. The child may be restless, delirious, and even hallucinate scary monsters or ghosts. *Belladonna* can bring improvement in as little as fifteen minutes.

Calcarea carbonica is good for some children with recurrent colds and ear infections, especially a baby with a big round head who sweats a lot and smells sour. They are chilly and sensitive to cold, yet they prefer ice cold drinks. They are chubby and placid. They are often allergic to milk.

Homeopathy can also be used at a deeper level for chronic, recurring problems, by strengthening the constitution. We are all born with certain hereditary factors that may predispose us to certain strengths or weaknesses of various organs and processes. Determining your child's constitutional type lets you know what his susceptibilities are. Administering the correct remedy in high potency can reprogram the human biocomputer and prevent a lifetime of misery.

MH's Story – ear infections

Thanks so much for helping me and my daughter for the last couple of years. It is long overdue, here are the highlights of the positive experiences we had with your treatment.
J used to have very dry hands in the winter. With Nat mur *(sodium chloride), her hands got better quickly. And, I remember one day after your* Sepia *remedy for J, her mood was better and she took the initiative to hug me for the first time in a long time.*
My ear infections were helped by Silica *and* Pulsatilla *almost immediately, although I did take a course of antibiotics for the last episode. But I believe the homeopathic remedy is the deciding factor to keep my ear totally clear and dry for quite a while now.*

Chapter 21

Homeopathy for Attention and Behavior Problems

Homeopathy is a medical science that uses remedies made from natural substances like plants and minerals to stimulate the body to heal itself. Besides curing acute illnesses, it works just as well for mental, emotional and behavioral problems, like ADD/ADHD, learning disability, emotional trauma, depression and anxiety. The choice of remedy is based on the symptoms, which are the body's way of telling you what it needs.

One of the most commonly needed remedies for Attention Deficit Hyperactivity Disorder (ADHD) is *Lycopodium*. Children who need this may be anxious, indecisive, timid and fearful of strangers, yet act like a bully to smaller children, or have a history of being bullied. They crave sweets and warm drinks, tend to have more problems on the right side of the body, sleep on their right side, and are tired or irritable after school, from around four pm to eight pm. Then they may get a second wind, and have trouble getting to sleep. They are also prone to dyslexia. They have a lot of digestive problems, including gassiness, especially after eating beans and vegetables of the cabbage family.

Polishing Diamonds

Nux vomica is for children who might be given a label of Oppositional Defiant Disorder (ODD). They are hyperactive, over excitable, and throw

134

tantrums when they don't get their way. They like to give orders
and blame others. They are rebels who need a cause. They are
oversensitive to noise, light, cold, odors, food, drugs, and being
awakened from a nap. They are also natural leaders, ambitious, highly
competitive, and determined to win. They are diamonds in the rough that
can be polished by homeopathy to bring out their natural brilliance and
remove the flaws.

Anxious Artists

Children needing *Phosphorus* have a lot of anxiety that "something may
happen", but can be easily reassured. They fear the dark, thunder,
spiders, and being alone. They are hypersensitive to their environment
and to the feelings of other people. They are very distractible, creative
and imaginative, and given to daydreaming. They would rather think
about having fun with their friends than pay attention in school, although
they are very intelligent. They are effervescent like the ice cold cola they
love to drink, have lots of friends, and often have musical or artistic
talents. Homeopathy can help them become more focused and able to
concentrate without interfering with their natural charm.

Smart but Shy

Silica is the remedy for children who are very shy, and afraid to try new
things because of fear of failure. They are very bright, but lack confidence
in themselves. Once they get up the courage to start something they will
do it well. They are said to lack "grit" and have trouble standing up for
themselves. They benefit from much encouragement. They can be
stubborn and set in their ways, but they won't argue or be aggressive.
They will just quietly do things in their own way. They are easily upset by
little things. They are content to live a quiet, low stress life in the slow
lane. Homeopathy can help them break through to a new level of
confidence, capability, self expression, and accomplishment.

Smart but Slow

135

Children who need the remedy *Calcaria carbonica* may be slower than average in development of mental and physical skills. They may be very intelligent, especially in highly structured fields like math and physics. They learn slowly but solidly. They have to fit every new piece of information into the right place in their body of knowledge, and they never forget it. They work hard and plod along, needing longer than others to finish their homework. They are not bored by repetition. They like sameness. They do not like changes in routine or plans. They are easily overwhelmed. They are very sensitive to criticism. They do not argue, probably because it would take too long to think of a good answer. When criticized, they withdraw into themselves, and in the future, may refuse to try. This may lead to lack of initiative and fear of failure even into adulthood. As an infant, this type looks like the Gerber baby, with a big round head. The head can get hot from mental effort, and sweats a lot, especially at night. They are picky eaters, and prefer bland food, like starches, eggs, and dairy products, which may not be good for them. They may be prone to celiac disease or lactose intolerance. They have a tendency to thyroid problems and gain weight easily. This is aggravated by their placid nature and dislike of physical activity. The remedy can help speed up normal development, and improve assimilation of calcium and other minerals needed for teeth, bones, nerves, skin and glands.

Too Good

Children who need the remedy *Natrum muriaticum* would not give anybody any problems, except themselves. They are very well behaved and obedient. They are overly serious, reserved, shy, sensitive, and self conscious. They may be insecure, obsessive, and perfectionistic, with a strong inner drive to succeed. They may have anxiety attacks before an exam. They shut down after the slightest criticism, and may go in their room, slam the door and cry alone. This is one of the best remedies for children suffering from depression, or grief from trauma, loss of a loved one, a grandparent's death, or parents' divorce, for which they may blame themselves. They may be introverted, preferring to stay home and read rather than go to parties. They don't have a lot of friends, but a few close ones. They like salty food and rainy days. They may get headaches from the sun and like to wear sunglasses. I have seen many children and adults emerge from sadness and grief after taking this remedy.

Curious Collectors

Sulfur is for the hyper in hyperactive, needed more often by boys than girls. They have immense energy and curiosity and have to touch everything. They have no fear of strangers, and ask endless questions about how everything works.   They even take things apart to see how they work. They are very messy and keep their room in total disorder. They collect things, and can't throw anything away. They love to wear old clothes until they're ragged, and think they're beautiful. They don't care about appearance, and hate to take a bath. They are self centered and need to be the center of attention. They interrupt and talk at length about what they are interested in, particularly areas of science, science fiction and fantasy. They often feel that rules don't apply to them. They assume leadership and organize group activities. They get high grades without studying much, procrastinate, and cram the night before a test. They start many things and don't finish, moving on to their next project. They are often considered lazy, except for their own interests. They spend more energy devising ways to avoid work than it would take to do the work. They may eventually benefit humanity by inventing labor saving devices. They are warm-blooded and define a sweater as "something I have to wear when my mother is cold". They like sweets, meat, and spicy food, and usually dislike vegetables. They get hungry at 11 a m and can't concentrate in the class before lunch. They are also prone to skin conditions like eczema and acne. A dose of *Sulfur* will bring out their good qualities and make life easier for the whole family as they grow up to fulfill their destiny.

Difficult Children

Some very difficult children who can be greatly benefitted by homeopathy are those who need *Tuberculinum*. These children have problems starting at birth, thought to be related to a history of tuberculosis in an ancestor.

They lag behind in milestones. They learn slowly, with difficult comprehension, poor concentration, and weak memory. They often end up in Special Education classes. They are extremely restless, with intense energy all day. They run, spin, and shout. Their sleep is restless, with grinding of teeth, sweats, and bed-wetting. They are irritable, especially on awakening, always dissatisfied and looking for change, wanting to move and travel. They can be malicious and violent, hitting, biting, cursing, and throwing things. They usually break things that others value the most. They may be self-destructive, throwing tantrums and banging their head on the floor. They may be violent toward animals, or have a fear of cats or dogs. They have weak lungs and are subject to chest ailments, colds, bronchitis, asthma, and chronic coughs, as well as recurrent ear infections. They may have chronic congestion from dairy products, although they crave cold milk. They may also have lactose intolerance and get diarrhea from milk.

These are only a few of the many homeopathic remedies that can be used to strengthen a child's constitution and improve their physical, mental, and emotional functioning. Homeopathy has no side effects, but when the remedy is given, the patient may feel worse before he feels better. Homeopathic remedies cure by presenting the body with an energy pattern which mimics the energy pattern of the disease, triggering exactly the correct healing response. Homeopathic remedies are so highly diluted that they contain no actual molecules of the original substance, only its energy pattern, or information.

DK's Story – ADD, etc.
Dr. Bonnie Camo has had a profound influence on my core beliefs about health in the close to thirty years that I've been her patient. I first met Dr. Camo when she was practicing with Dr. Pfeiffer at what was then the Princeton Brain Bio Center in New Jersey. The Center and the doctors who worked there in the early 80's were amazing and people came from all over the country to have their blood work done and to get nutritional solutions to their health problems.

Dr. Camo left the Center shortly after Dr. Pfeiffer's death and I followed her practice. Once she became licensed in homeopathy she added that component to her practice and I began to learn about homeopathy in addition to nutrition through her.

Other members of my family went to her as well. When my nephew, who was seven years old, was diagnosed by doctors out in his home state of New Mexico with ADD and given a prescription for Ritalin—my sister brought my nephew to Dr. Camo who found, after a blood test, that excess lead was the culprit to his hyperactivity, and prescribed a nutritional supplement (molybdenum) to help clear the lead out of his system rather than the Ritalin.

When I suffered from severe eczema, Dr. Camo prescribed Borage oil and a variety of other supplements rather than put me on a life-long program of cortisone which the local dermatologist prescribed. She helped me understand allergies and taught me about the importance of a food rotation diet.

Her non-invasive approach has been a comfort and a gift to me. No radical diagnosis, no harmful drugs—just balanced and sound nutritional advice backed up with research.

Dr. Camo has also helped my parents, who are now in their 80's, through the ups and downs of aging. She has supported their good health through homeopathy and nutritional supplementation which has kept them active and healthy all these years. I know that her calm and balanced approach has saved me and my parents a lot of white coat anxiety.

The world would be a cleaner and healthier place if there were more doctors like Dr. Camo.

I encourage all who read Dr. Camo's advice in this book to take heart in knowing that they have discovered one of the all-time greats. A genuinely nutritionally-oriented physician who has spent a lifetime helping people get healthy naturally and without harmful side effects. She is one of the best doctors I have had the pleasure to know in this life and I am so thankful that I have had the good fortune of having her as a guiding light for all these years.

Chapter 22

Homeopathy for Depression

It is normal to feel grief and sadness after suffering a loss, such as death of a loved one, financial set-backs, illness, infirmity or aging that render people unable to do things they used to enjoy. These conditions are not diseases that need to be treated with drugs. Using pharmaceuticals to treat unpleasant life events can turn sadness into legal drug addiction. It is easy for a psychiatrist to put suffering people on these drugs; they know no other way to treat. Although it is claimed that these drugs are not addictive, it is very difficult for people to get off them. Anti-depressants have numerous side effects, such as weight gain, loss of interest in sex, even suicide, especially in young people. Teenagers and younger and younger children are being given labels of depression and bipolar disorder and put on drugs that have never even been tested on children. When people try to get off these drugs, their depression often comes back worse than ever, along with other symptoms they never had before being put on antidepressants. And as previously discussed, these drugs don't even work; many studies show they are no better than placebos.

Cure for a Broken Heart

If sadness is too severe or lingers too long, it can easily be treated with homeopathy. There are remedies for ailments from a broken heart."Physical symptoms of grief ", as my teacher Dr. Luc de Schepper called them, include cravings for salty things, thirst for cold drinks, sensation of a lump in the throat, cold sore flare-ups, dry skin and lips, loss of appetite,
headaches or eye pain from sunlight. People with this type of depression

tend to suppress their feelings and are usually unable to cry, except perhaps at sad movies or when alone in their room.   Many of my patients with these symptoms, even years after a sad event, have been helped by the remedy *Natrum muriaticum*, made from sodium chloride, table salt. The remedy often brings up sad memories that have been repressed, and then they will cry and feel much better. For more acute grief symptoms, with shock, disbelief, hysteria, sighing, sobbing, and mood swings, *Ignatia* may bring welcome relief.

Gold for Loss of Gold!

Depression due to business failure, financial loss and bankruptcy is becoming more common, with the current economic situation in this country and the world. After the stock market crashes of 1929 and 1987,(both in October), many victims who lost their fortunes went into deep depression, even committing suicide. Before their devastating losses, such people had often been intense, idealistic, and goal oriented, wanting and achieving the best. With frustration of their goals they became subject to irritability and anger.   With loss of meaning in their life, many became vulnerable to alcohol or addictions, perhaps in an attempt to fill their deep spiritual longings. The remedy for this type of depression is actually gold! Ironically, the metal gold, symbol and source of wealth and security, in homeopathic form, *Aurum metallicum*, often brings relief from suicidal depression due to loss of financial security. It may also relieve depression from loss of emotional security, after the death of their lifelong companion.

Post-Partum Depression

Symptoms of hypothyroidism frequently begin after giving birth, resulting in depression, irritability, weight gain, fatigue, and loss of sex drive. Women in this situation are very sensitive to cold and actually have a lower than normal body temperature and low blood pressure. They feel much better with vigorous exercise or dancing that raises their blood pressure and increases their body temperature up closer to 98.6degrees, which is

optimum for all chemical reactions in the body. These women will benefit from the homeopathic remedy *Sepia*, made from the ink of the sepia squid. Although most often needed by women, this remedy was first used by Hahnemann to treat a man, a depressed artist who used squid ink to paint sepia-toned paintings. The artist used his lips to make a point on his brush, thus ingesting squid ink and "proving" the remedy, the same one Hahnemann used, in homeopathic form, to cure his depression.

People Who Need People

People who need the remedy *Phosphorus* are usually in good spirits, very friendly, open and sympathetic. They can literally feel other people's pain and suffering. They often feel that they are psychic or clairvoyant, and can have precognitive dreams. They only sleep on their right side, because they feel their heart palpitating if they try to sleep on the left. Many artists and musically talented people fall into this group. They can be very emotional and melodramatic, magnifying minor symptoms into fear of serious disease, but are very easily reassured by their doctor. They are people who need people, and can get depressed when they are alone, or if they overload themselves with activities and burn out. Although chilly and sensitive to cold, they tend to have a great craving for ice cold drinks, especially colas , which, ironically, contain phosphorus, in the form of phosphoric acid.

Placid Plodders

A tendency to low thyroid function in childhood is more common in people with Type O blood, and may be helped by homeopathy. *Calcaria carbonica*, made from calcium carbonate, or oyster shell, is a remedy that often benefits children of this type, who are said to be oyster-like in their tendency to be sedentary and placid. They have low energy, gain weight easily, and suffer from the cold, but sweat a lot on the head at night. Their susceptibility to colds, sore throats, and ear infections often improves when dairy products are avoided. Once they have been treated with *Calc carb*,

142

their energy and resistance to infection improve, and they may also be better able to tolerate milk products.

Fear of Speaking

Lycopodium is a remedy for people who don't "like a podium". This is a little joke I make to help people remember the name of their remedy, because their greatest fear is public speaking. They fear meeting new people and any new situation. They may have a fear of responsibility and commitment. Males of this type may prefer one night stands to a committed relationship, or may have problems with impotence. They are socially awkward, lack courage, and suffer from feelings of inadequacy. Their energy is lowest in late afternoon, classically from 4 to 8 pm. They tend to have more problems on the right side of their body.

Weepy Wilter

A depressed woman needing the remedy *Pulsatilla* is very emotional and expresses her feelings openly, easily breaking into gentle weeping. She feels forsaken and benefits from much attention and consolation. She has difficulty being independent and standing up for herself, and making decisions. She is very feminine, mild-tempered and agreeable, and often feels most fulfilled in life by being a good wife and a loving mother. She may crave creamy foods and peanut butter, and wilts in hot weather.

Depression is often caused by grief, from loss of a loved one, romantic disappointment, setbacks in life, losses, or just a realistic appraisal of the current world situation. The climate crisis, destruction of nature, impending financial collapse, epidemics, etc may lead one to say, "If you're not depressed, you're not paying attention". But depression leads to apathy, and today we need all the energy we can muster just to survive. Homeopathy is extremely useful to help a person recover from misfortunes, to help reverse an overly pessimistic outlook, and to strengthen the constitution to better withstand the inevitable stresses of life.

SM's story – depression and negativity
Being the logical person I am, who would think I would have begun believing my boyfriend knew my future and had psychic powers that would terrify me. But this is how it went for me, before I was old enough to know what I was experiencing and how to deal with it. This experience just became a part of my reality; and only a person who experiences a perceptual shift like this can even imagine what that is like. Anyhow, as time elapsed, the strange and scary thoughts subsided. Although, I knew I wasn't alright.   So I saw a therapist and that didn't help. Then I bought some self-help books and started exercising daily and repeating positive affirmations to myself. But as time wore on nothing brought me back to feeling my usual happy-go-lucky self. I didn't recognize myself in many ways.
 Six months later, you could say I had what a psychiatrist would call "negative symptoms."   I wasn't feeling much emotion, nor did I feel comfortable being around anyone.   A lot of stimuli caused me to become totally overwhelmed, so I avoided many "normal" situations. I didn't really know what I was feeling, thinking, and surely couldn't find my own internal drive for anything. In short, I was lost. From that time forward, I remained lost for several years to come, despite the efforts of psychiatrists who gave me antidepressants, then later antipsychotics and mood stabilizing medications.
 None of this helped me to feel myself and I became so desperate after six years of unsuccessful treatment, I went to Earth House. [a half-way house for young people with schizophrenia and other mental illnesses, that uses nutritional therapy along with medication. -BC] *At this point, I was fat. I had gained sixty pounds in three months as a result of taking anti-psychotic drugs. These drugs mentally lobotomized me and in retrospect were the most barbaric excuse for a "medicine" I could ever imagine encountering.   Nevertheless, Earth House's approach was a welcomed contrast having a focus on vitamins, nutrition, therapy, exercise, and homeopathy in treating mental illness.   This place was a beacon of hope for me. Was it possible I could retrieve my identity and peace of mind after all this time? I once had had a strong personality as a young girl and didn't know if I would ever return to normal.*
It wasn't until I began to see Dr. Camo for homeopathic remedies that I felt I was making any 'real' progress.   These remedies internally changed me

but not in a synthetic way, like how medications made me feel. From 1998 forward, I have accomplished getting two master's degrees, and a massage therapy license. Now I am a professor and feel I owe much of my success to having taken homeopathic remedies. I'm not saying it has been easy, just that this was the best solution I could come up with; certainly better than pharmaceutical drugs. I also realize homeopathy doesn't receive attention as a viable form of treatment because it is not lucrative. No expensive pills!!! Anyhow, I'd recommend homeopathy with a supplement of vitamins and exercise to anyone struggling with mental illness as the best possible mode of treatment.

Chapter 23
Homeopathy for Anxiety, Fear, and Phobias

Many homeopathic remedies are made from highly poisonous plants and other deadly substances like snake venom. The more severe symptoms a substance can cause, the more severe the symptoms it can relieve. An example of this is the remedy *Aconitum*, made from a relative of Delphinium, often grown in ornamental flower gardens. Aconite, also known as monkshood and wolfsbane, was historically used to poison wolves. If the plant is eaten by mistake, symptoms of poisoning occur very rapidly, after only a few minutes, starting with numbness of the tongue and mouth, nausea, and vomiting. The numbness then spreads until it covers the skin of the entire body, along with the sensation of burning and of ants crawling on the skin, and extreme coldness, like ice water running in the veins. Color vision may be reduced to yellow and green, and there may be ringing in the ears, and eventually, after a half hour to three hours, paralysis of the limbs and finally the heart. Naturally anyone in this situation would be seized with extreme fear. Hahnemann used reports of poisoning in the literature to help him understand the conditions that a remedy might be used to treat.

Aconitum is the number one remedy for shock and intense fear that comes on suddenly, such as after a car accident or natural disaster or other frightening experience. It is also good for severe anxiety and panic attacks, with tremendous terror of dying or feeling that death is imminent. The person may even predict the time of death. There may be hyperventilation, palpitations, dry mouth, flushed face or pallor. The symptoms, whether due to actual frightening causes or psychological disorders, come on very suddenly and with great intensity. The remedy is even effective years after a frightening event, which the person has never gotten over, so it can be helpful for post-traumatic stress disorder (PTSD).

The Perfectionist

Arsenicum may benefit people who live in a state of chronic anxiety and insecurity, fearing loss of money, possessions, health and their very life. They have a tremendous fear of death or developing a chronic disease like cancer. Their fear of disease leads them to a fear of germs and extreme fastidiousness, even to becoming a compulsive cleaner or "neat freak". They save everything, carefully organized and labeled (in contrast to *Sulfur* people, who save everything in a disorganized mess.) Fear of losing their wealth and property makes them very selfish and self centered. They can be obsessive and compulsive as they try to get control over their environment in order to feel more secure. They are afraid to be alone and need a strong support network. They are dependent on their family and friends and so have great anxiety for their well-being.

Stage Fright

Gelsemium is a great remedy for stage fright, as well as for fear of going to a doctor or dentist, dread of traveling by plane, nervousness before taking exams, and anticipatory anxiety before any type of performance or ordeal. There may be diarrhea or trembling from fear, anticipation, or hearing bad news. The person feels weak and timid and lacks confidence. *Gelsemium* has even been used to treat cowardice on the battlefield.

Fear of Getting Lost

People who need *Lycopodium* also suffer from anticipatory anxiety, especially if they have to give a speech, or speak in front of the class in school. They may put on a courageous front and bluff their way through. Once they actually begin speaking, they usually do okay. *Lycopodium* people may also have a fear of getting lost or being unable to reach their destination, literally or metaphorically.

Superstitious

Argentum nitricum is another remedy for anticipatory anxiety. People who will benefit from this also have a fear of heights, because they may have an impulse to jump. They also have impulses to do other dangerous things that they are afraid they may carry out. They fear looking up at tall buildings, which they think may fall on them. They may have a fear of driving, especially over bridges.   They are very superstitious and may develop compulsive thoughts and behavior.

Fear of Animals

Certain remedy types have fears of various animals or insects. *Calcaria carbonica* has a fear of mice and rats. *Lachesis* (made from snake venom), *Natrum muriaticum* and *Lac caninum* all have a fear of snakes. *Belladonna* has a fear of dogs, especially black dogs. *Tuberculinum* has a fear of cats. *Phosphorus* has a fear of spiders and insects, (and also a big fear of thunderstorms).   *Ignatia* has a fear of birds or chickens.

MH's Story – fear of driving
For myself, the most dramatic experience was with Silica. *After the first dose in your office, I was driving home on Route 18 inner left lane naturally without any fear! I was always afraid of driving on the left lanes ever since I had a car accident years ago.*

Chapter 24

Homeopathy for Anger, Irritability and Rage

Nux vomica is for the "Type A" personality, very intense, irritable, driven, ambitious and competitive. They are very impatient and can't stand waiting in line or in traffic. They can dish it out but they can't take it. Easily offended and angered by contradiction, they may break or throw things when angry. They are very sensitive to noise, light, odors, and especially being awakened from a nap. They may crave coffee, drugs and alcohol. *Nux* is also the main remedy for hangovers.

Pre-Menstrual Syndrome

People who need *Sepia* are usually women, who have a lot of anger and irritability, along with their depression. All of this is aggravated premenstrually. They become more and more detached and indifferent to their family and community. They lose their temper, yell and scream when confronted by their children's demands, and just want to be left alone. The best way for them to cope and get back to normal is to go out for a run or go to a gym for a vigorous workout.

Angry Infants

Chamomilla is a remedy often needed by angry children and infants. They want to be carried or rocked all the time. They are very capricious, asking for things and then throwing them away. Their crying has a very irritating quality that makes parents want to hit them to shut them up. (In contrast, *Pulsatilla* types have a gentle weeping that makes you want to console them, which they love.) *Chamomillas* are very sensitive to pain and shriek angrily if touched where it hurts. It is the classic remedy for teething pain in infants.

Belladonna is a remedy for sudden, intense, violent, aggressive rage, with shrieking, hitting, biting, spitting, head-banging, and hair pulling, which may be caused by a fever, drug-induced delirium, mania or acute psychosis. The face is bright red and hot, with dilated pupils and wild, staring eyes, as the person may be undergoing vivid, frightening hallucinations.

Stramonium is another remedy for violent, delirious, destructive rage that comes in outbursts, almost like a convulsion, with cursing, laughing, screaming and biting. It may be precipitated by meningitis, head injury, epilepsy, or witnessing acts of violence. It is accompanied by extreme fear, nightmares or night terrors, and fear of the dark, dogs, water, and shiny surfaces like mirrors.

Nitricum acidum is needed by some people with a very negative, pessimistic personality. They are prone to extreme irritability, especially on waking in the morning. They are often involved in quarrels with family members, neighbors or coworkers that can go on for years, and are "unmoved by apologies". They tend to be very selfish and feel that other people are the same way. They are also extremely anxious about their health. *Nit ac* has been described as the most hypochondriacal remedy in the entire Materia Medica. They fear cancer, AIDS and death itself. They are likely to accuse their homeopath of making them worse, and even if they feel better, are reluctant to admit it. They tend to be very chilly, and crave fat and salt.

Cystitis and Anger

Cantharis is generally thought of as one of the leading remedies for cystitis, with a rapid onset of severe burning pain on urination. It also helps burning pain in the eyes, throat, stomach and elsewhere, from various pathologies. The mental state is one of great anger and irritability, even violent rage and delirium. I recall a young woman I was seeing for a diagnosis of schizophrenia, who had a very negative, angry attitude that switched to friendly and cooperative immediately after I gave her a dose of *Cantharis* for a bladder infection. It was amazing. And I had a student with me at the time to verify her remarkable sudden turnaround.

Chapter 25
Homeopathy for Women's Problems

Puberty can be a difficult time for boys as well as girls, but girls have the additional problem of waiting for the periods to start. A girl can be embarrassed if she is the first among her peers to start, but it is even worse if her menarche is late, with a general delay in development of breasts and pubic hair. Delayed puberty can be caused by nutritional deficiencies, anorexia or excessive dieting, (which seems to be starting at younger and younger ages), as well as the growing problem of obesity in children.

Pulsatilla is a major remedy for problems that begin around the time of puberty. Its picture of moodiness, weepiness and irritability fits the state of mind of a young girl with delay in onset and establishment of regular cycles, especially if she seems somewhat immature, timid, and passive. If periods are delayed into the late teens, *Natrum muriaticum* may be helpful, especially in a girl who is overly serious or may have suffered from emotional trauma, such as losing a loved one or breaking up with a boyfriend.

PMS Remedies

PMS or premenstrual syndrome responds well to homeopathy, avoiding the need for Prozac-like drugs under other names for this common

154

condition, now known by more serious sounding names like PMDD (Premenstrual Dysphoric Disorder.) Along with irritability or weepiness, there may be breast swelling and tenderness and general fluid retention. *Natrum muriaticum* is one of the best remedies if there is marked fluid

retention, aggravated by a craving for salt, depression with desire to be alone, and migraines preceded by flickering zigzags in the visual field.

A woman needing *Sepia* for PMS will be irritable and angry, especially at her husband, and totally uninterested in sex, which may even be painful. She is likely to scream at the children at this time, and wants to get away from the whole family. She may crave sweets or sour food, rather than salt, and may also develop premenstrual migraines.

The *Nux vomica* woman is also irritable and angry, and may be even more of a workaholic than usual. She is likely to be constipated with ineffectual urging and crampy, spasmodic pain, frequent urination and chilliness.

In a woman needing *Lachesis*, all symptoms will be worse on awakening from sleep, worse on the left side of the body, and she will be unable to tolerate tight clothing, especially around the neck. As soon as the bleeding starts, all symptoms will quickly resolve.

The fatigue, weakness, and self-consciousness of a *Calcaria carbonica* woman will be aggravated premenstrually. She may lose her appetite or have a craving for sweets or eggs. She may be chillier than usual, with itching and sweating in the genital area.

Help for Infertility

Infertility seems to be becoming more and more common, perhaps due to the hormone-disrupting chemicals now flooding our environment, like pesticides and plastics. Sperm counts have decreased by fifty percent in recent decades, according to Theo Colborn, et al in <u>Our Stolen Future</u>.

Eating a healthy diet of organic vegetables, fruits, and protein sources would be a good prerequisite before attempting pregnancy. Taking their particular constitutional remedies will help both partners achieve their goal.

Agnus castus is a useful remedy for infertility with weak ovarian function and general weakness and lack of interest in sex. It also helps impotence in the male. *Lycopodium* is helpful when the right fallopian tube or ovary has been damaged by previous inflammation, or cysts on the right ovary. It also helps impotence and premature ejaculation in the male. *Sepia* helps both genders with weak libido and low sexual interest.

Morning Nausea

There is a whole field of gynecological homeopathy to help in pregnancy and delivery. One of the most useful remedies for morning sickness is *Pulsatilla*, with intolerance of heat and aversion to greasy or fatty food. The nausea may be in the afternoon or evening as well as morning, and changes from day to day. There is little thirst, except perhaps for cold lemonade. As usual with this remedy there is weepiness, timidity and passivity.

Sepia is another big remedy for morning sickness, which may be worse around 3 to 5 pm. There may or may not be loss of appetite, but the woman feels better after eating. Vomiting is followed by exhaustion or fatigue, and constipation. There is a dragging or empty feeling in the abdomen, and the mood is one of irritability or indifference.

The woman who needs *Sulfur* for nausea of pregnancy has a sour, burning vomit with an offensive odor, which may occur soon after eating. There is great hunger, and often diarrhea on awakening.

For recurrent miscarriages, *Pulsatilla* and *Sepia* are again useful, with the usual accompanying symptoms of these remedies. *Sabina* is another remedy that can prevent as well as treat recurrent miscarriage around the twelfth week. There may be pain in the kidney area and thighs, and great sensitivity to heat.

Caulophyllum is one of the most important remedies for the actual delivery, especially where there is poor muscle tone, contractions are

short and irregular, and the cervix fails to dilate. *Arnica* is always good for the bruising and soreness after delivery. *Staphysagria* is important to help heal the episiotomy, or the incision for a cesarean delivery.

Post-partum depression with rejection of the husband and even the baby will usually respond to *Sepia*, which will also help restore sexual desire which is often lost after birth of a baby. If there is hopeless despair and suicidal feelings, *Aurum* may benefit. For milder sadness with changeable mood, desire for company, thirstlessness, and intolerance of heat, *Pulsatilla* will be the remedy.

Menopause

Menopausal symptoms can be greatly alleviated by homeopathy. *Sepia* is again one of the most commonly used remedies, as it helps relieve hormonal imbalances. It addresses hot flashes, faint feelings, anxiety, and loss of interest in sex. It is indicated for a bearing down sensation, as if everything will fall out through the vagina, as well as for actual prolapse of the uterus. The woman often sits with her legs tightly crossed, as if to prevent anything falling out.

Lachesis is another important remedy for menopause, with hot flashes, fainting, weakness, uterine cramps, and profuse sweating. All symptoms are worse after sleep, and mainly on the left side, such as headaches and ovarian pain. She tends to be jealous and suspicious, and retains her strong sex drive.

A menopausal woman needing *Natrum muriaticum* becomes increasingly introverted and has difficulty expressing her feelings. She is depressed, tense and irritable, and wants to be alone. Like *Sepia*, she has a tendency to uterine prolapse, as well as dryness of the vagina, so she also has little interest in sex. She may actually feel better on a rainy day.

Pulsatilla has milder hot flashes, aggravated by hot weather. She expresses her emotions easily, with rapid changes in mood, and cries openly when she feels like it.

Sulfur is for a woman who may feel hot all the time after menopause, but still has hot flashes, preceded by shivering. She may become less interested in personal hygiene, bathing less frequently and wanting to wear old comfortable clothes.

What about Hormones?

In addition to homeopathy to control their distressing symptoms, many menopausal women may be wondering about taking hormones. Hormone replacement therapy for menopausal women is an ongoing dilemma. Every few years new studies are done, usually giving results contradicting previous studies, so women are put on and taken off of postmenopausal hormones.

Estrogen had been promoted as preventing heart disease, osteoporosis and Alzheimer's disease, but was then found to increase the risk of uterine and breast cancer. "Progesterone" was supposed to mitigate the risk of uterine cancer caused by estrogen, but could increase the risk of other types of cancer.

One of the causes of all this confusion is that the studies are not done with actual bioidentical hormones (the same as what the human body makes), but with estrogen taken from pregnant horses (which is different from human estrogen), and synthetic unnatural analogs of progesterone, known as progestins. These are totally different from natural bioidentical progesterone, cannot be broken down by the body's metabolic pathways, and may interfere with the body's own progesterone.

Bioidentical progesterone can be made from the Mexican yam (Dioscorea), but this conversion cannot be performed in the human body, so "yam creams" sold in health food stores for menopausal problems are probably useless. Creams containing natural progesterone are also sold over the counter, and are useful for premenstrual syndrome, menopausal symptoms, and prevention of osteoporosis, according to the research of Dr. John Lee.

Bioidentical estrogen has been popularized by people like actress Suzanne Somers, who apparently cured her breast cancer by using natural substances, while taking bioidentical estrogen. Three forms of estrogen are made by the human body: estrone, estradiol and estriol. Estriol is the weakest, has a cancer-preventing effect, and is probably safest to use for menopausal symptoms, especially vaginal dryness, in the form of a vaginal cream available from compounding pharmacies. Conventional doctors are not yet convinced of the value of bioidentical hormones, but doctors familiar with alternative and natural medicine can perform tests using blood or saliva and prescribe natural estrogens, progesterone, and testosterone if needed, formulated to your exact needs by compounding pharmacies.

Cystitis

Homeopathy is also beneficial for infections to which women are susceptible, such as bladder infections, or cystitis. The conventional approach is to treat with antibiotics, which will replace a bladder infection with a yeast infection. The most commonly needed remedy for acute cystitis is *Cantharis*, which relieves burning pain before, during or after urination, as well as urgency and frequency. *Sarsaparilla* can be considered for severe burning pain after urination, and constant urging.

Equisitum is for a constant feeling of bladder fullness and tenderness, not relieved by urination. There may be some incontinence, especially at night. (This remedy is also good for bedwetting in children.) There may be burning, prickling pain in the urethra during or after urination. Antibiotics given for cystitis or other infections may kill off the body's natural "good" bacteria along with the "bad" ones, resulting in overgrowth of yeast organisms such as Candida. This can result in digestive upsets as well as a vaginal yeast infection.   Probiotics such as acidophilus or yogurt with active cultures can help restore normal flora. Homeopathic remedies such as *Sepia* and *Pulsatilla* can work wonders, as well as a remedy made from *Candida*, the disease organism itself, a form of homeopathy known as isopathy.

Chapter 26

Homeopathy for First Aid and Natural Disasters

In summertime, many of us spend a lot of time in the outdoors, subject to nature's slings and arrows, bee stings, bug bites, bumps and bruises, sunburn, poison ivy, etc. Homeopathy can mitigate all of these minor disasters, as well as travel-associated maladies like motion sickness and jet lag. Even victims of major disasters, such as earthquakes and hurricanes, could benefit from homeopathy, which is cheap, effective, and has no side effects.

The premier homeopathic first aid remedy, which many people are already familiar with, is *Arnica montana, Arnica* for short. This is a made from a daisy that grows in mountainous areas of Europe, where it is known locally by names like Bruisewort and Fall Herb, by virtue of its ability to relieve effects of falls and other injuries. It was also known to the Native American Indians. Its value as a vulnerary (wound healer) has been known since ancient times. I have used it innumerable times myself. I once ran a screwdriver through my thumbnail while trying to fix a broken window crank. I put a few pellets on my tongue and the excruciating pain was relieved instantly! Another time a poorly installed cupboard came loose from the wall and fell on my forehead, producing a lump the size of half an egg. I took *Arnica* and by next morning the swelling was gone and it was as if I had never been injured.

162

Arnica is the first remedy to take after any injury or trauma. I always carry some in my purse. Thirty c or 200c are good potencies to use. It is useful for overuse or strain of any organ, such as excessive gardening or yard work. It is also good for jetlag and that tired, bruised feeling after a long car or plane ride, while trying to sleep in odd positions. (Another thing that helps jet lag is gazing at a sunset or sunrise in your new location so the body knows how to orient itself in time and space.)

I used to be subject to car sickness as a child and air sickness as an adult. There are two main remedies for this: *Cocculus* and *Tabacum* (made from tobacco). Hopefully none of you readers are smokers, but if any of you ever tried it, you may remember how your first puff caused nausea, giddiness, a deathly sinking feeling, icy coldness and sweats, very similar to how I used to feel on a plane, especially when it circles around and around, waiting to land. Taking a dose of *Tabacum* an hour before takeoff and landing prevents this. For some people, *Cocculus* may work better, for vertigo and dizziness with nausea and vomiting, fear, fatigue and loss of sleep.

For bee stings, or anything that causes burning, stinging, redness and swelling, especially if it feels worse from heat and better from cool applications, the remedy is *Apis*, made from honey bee venom. It is also good for allergic reactions to bee or wasp stings. For bug bites, even tick bites, and puncture wounds, *Ledum* may help, especially if the wounded parts feel cold. If given immediately after puncture wounds, it prevents tetanus, according to Robin Murphy, in <u>Lotus Materia Medica</u>. In case of splinters, *Silica* may help expel them from the body. I had a patient with a piece of glass imbedded in her back, from a fall onto a lamp. After taking *Silica*, the glass came out.

For sunburn, *Urtica urens*, made from stinging nettle, is a good choice, for intense burning, itching and vesicles. (A non-homeopathic remedy for sunburn or any burn is Aloe vera gel applied directly onto the burned area. Keep a jar of it by the stove, or break a leaf from a live Aloe vera plant on your windowsill.)

For that summertime scourge poison ivy, a homeopathic dose of poison ivy leaf, *Rhus toxicodendron*, may prove to you that like cures like. A 200c or higher dose works best. It is also good for any rash that looks like poison ivy, with redness, swelling, and intense itching, ameliorated by heat. *Rhus tox* is also well known as one of the best remedies for arthritis, rheumatism, and fibromyalgia.

Aconite is used for effects of severe anxiety, fright and shock, and emotional trauma. It benefits victims of accidents and natural disasters, along with *Arnica* for the physical trauma. *Aconite* is also good for injuries to the eye.

RM's Story –tendonitis

These two success stories [previously described - BC] *prompted me to write a letter to the Princeton Brain Bio Center on April 26, 1984, to ask if they accepted patients for preventive medicine. They did, and I have been going to them, or you, every year since 1984. I was 39 then, am 62 now, have been taking your vitamins and minerals the entire time and have been healthy the entire time.*

Once I came to you complaining of "mouse elbow" (I am an old computer programmer). I had initially gone to a local doctor who made the diagnosis (tendonitis) but whose cure did not work. He gave me a pain killer which only masked the symptoms and cured nothing, and he had me wear an Ace bandage with also did nothing. When I told you about it on my next regular visit, you gave me the homeopathic treatment of Ruta. *Within ten days my right elbow was fine and has been ever since. (I am more careful about how and how much I use the mouse now.)*

About five years ago I was diagnosed with ulnar nerve entrapment in my left elbow, again from excessive computer use. I went to local doctors who did nerve conductance and other tests. They said that surgery might be necessary but they would try to treat it without surgery first. Their

164

surgeon told me that vitamin B-6 was excellent for regrowing nerve

sheathing and said I should up my daily dose to 400mg per day. He also prescribed "nerve glide" exercises and other physical therapy. The condition was treated successfully without surgery but I found it very interesting that a surgeon would recommend vitamin therapy. He said "the best surgery is no surgery."

LF's story -- food reaction
I recall one evening, having dinner at Dr. Camo's, at one point my wife, S, became glassy-eyed and lethargic. We did not know the cause, but surmised that it might have been something she ate, which produced an allergic reaction. Bonnie left the room and returned with a small vial containing a homeopathic remedy [histaminum- BC]. A few moments after ingesting the remedy, S was wide awake, alert, and asking what happened. I was happy to have experienced this dramatic, positive reaction first hand.

BB's story – Reflections on My Homeopathic Experiences

During my childhood, I had been taken to a homeopathic doctor for various illnesses, frequent colds, and the mandatory school vaccinations. When he retired, I didn't see any doctors on a regular basis for many years except for surgery, earaches, delivering babies, and occasional falls or injuries. Finally I found Dr. Bonnie Camo, and my health began to improve as I recognized the taste of the familiar little white homeopathic pellets. Reflecting on my experiences with homeopathy over the years, I see that I have had an assortment of homeopathic remedies for various symptoms and conditions.
Recently, after a rainy summer, and no chance to work in my garden, I did a seven-hour marathon of weeding. I didn't think of anything past getting a hot shower that night. The next morning, my muscles were seized up and I could hardly move for the next ten days. Once I recovered, I was again weeding the garden, this time for only five

hours. On taking my shower, I reflected that I again would probably be immobile for days. I thought of Arnica and took a dose after my shower, and again the next morning and evening, for several days. Bruising and sore muscles were kept at bay this time, and I am sure that I will remember to turn to Arnica in the future.

Arnica helped to hasten my healing for "the most serious surgery a human being can undergo" (in the words of my surgeon). In this surgery, two-thirds of my pancreas, my spleen, and gallbladder were removed, along with a basketball-sized serous cystadenoma which was, thank God, benign. It was very serious for I remember dying, and being sent back (because I "have a lot of work to do"), and waking up three days after the surgery.

Once they realized that I was awake, I had to get out of bed onto a chair, and then, when I didn't fall over, was asked to "walk to the door"! When I had satisfied all requests and was left sitting alone, I went to my room-locker, got out my Arnica, and took my first post-operative dose. In the following week, I continued taking the Arnica. My doctors and nurses were amazed at how nicely I was progressing. They noted on my chart that I was "taking homeopathic remedies". Although this was such major surgery, with a large incision, I had minimal bruising. Arnica has, time and again, proven itself worthy of a permanent place in my home remedy kit.

After my surgery, I began to mis-write words (i.e., starting writing a word from the middle, then adding the first few letters, even as I saw it was wrong from the beginning). Lycopodium took care of that in short order, much to my relief.

Silica also has proven itself to me to be a reliable remedy. After a fall on broken milk glass, Silica came to the rescue to draw out pieces of glass shards, as well as the rose thorn-tips embedded in my arms after pruning out dead branches. Silica has also made me voice my opinions and speak up for myself in situation where, formerly, I had inwardly fumed in silence at being taken advantage of and being put upon by those who expected me to sacrifice my own time and well-being at their whims and wishes.

Rhus tox cured a bad case of poison ivy in a few days, and although I have been near it since, so far I have not had a recurrence. Of course, I look out for it, and I avoid touching it too.

During dental work, when I had been given a large dose of Novocain, I suffered a sensation of my skin burning, starting at the site of the injection and spreading over my face, scalp, and neck, down my arms, chest, and back to my waist. One dose of Cantharis *relieved the burning; it reversed its course, and was gone in a few days.* Cantharis *also helped for a stubborn urinary tract infection, along with (sugar free) cranberry juice.*

A near-collision with an SUV, whose driver was more intent on using his cell phone than paying attention that he was speeding and crossing three lanes without looking, caused me to floor my brakes and make a sudden stop. I was extremely upset and couldn't sleep. A dose of Aconite *helped me so that I felt all the hairs on my body relax from head to toe. I finally felt calmer and slept all weekend. I alternated* Arnica *(for my bruises and injuries from flooring my brakes) and* Aconite *for a week and felt much calmer, finally letting go of the intense fear of what surely would have been a fatal collision.*

When I lost my mother, followed six weeks later by my former husband and friend, followed by five other life-long friends and my teacher within eighteen months, I was overcome by a deep numbing grief. Nat mur *has helped me through this difficult time. Although I still grieve some, it is receding with time.*

I have taken other homeopathic remedies over the years such as Lycopodium, Sepia, Sulphur, *and others. All had a turn and helped me over whatever was the "crisis of the moment".*

After this reflection on some of my remedies, it would be difficult to say which one I would choose if I could only be allowed to keep one in my remedy kit, but if pushed, I must choose Arnica. *For injury, shock, serious surgery, and sore muscles from overexertion and gardening,* Arnica *has been my "go to" first line of relief. I now reach for it whenever I finish my gardening exertions. Weeding has lost its bite.*

Homeopathy works, and I am grateful to have a natural way to keep healthy. I only have to say that I will miss seeing Dr. Camo since she is retiring. She has taught me so much about homeopathic remedies and how to use them to help myself keep healthy naturally.

Part 4

Environment and Health

Chapter 27

Light and Health

All life on earth evolved under the natural light of the sun, with its full spectrum of wavelengths which we see as the colors of the rainbow. Many ancient peoples and civilizations worshiped the sun as the source of life and healing powers. Ancient Egypt worshiped the sun god Ra in various forms during the millennia of its history.   Heliopolis, Greek for "city of the sun", was a city in ancient Egypt widely known for its temples of healing, where sunlight was broken up into its component spectrum of colors.   Each color was used for a specific medical problem. Herodotus, the father of heliotherapy, treatment by sunlight, wrote that "exposure to the sun is highly necessary in persons whose health needs restoring." (<u>Light: Medicine of the Future</u>   Jacob Liberman, 1991)

Before Thomas Edison invented the electric light bulb in 1879, people spent most of their time outdoors, and received adequate daily doses of natural full spectrum sunlight.   Today most of us spend most of our lives indoors, under artificial lights. We are told not to go out without sunscreen lotions and special sunglasses. We are taught that the sun is our enemy, full of deadly ultraviolet.

What is Ultraviolet?

Sunlight contains the whole spectrum of wavelengths, or frequencies, that our eyes perceive as color. The shortest wavelengths are seen as violet (400 nanometers), progressively lengthening through blue, green, yellow and orange to red, (750 nm) the longest. Waves longer than red, known as infra red, are not seen, but felt as heat. The shortest wavelength human eyes can see is violet. But other animals, including bees, can see the shorter ultraviolet waves that are invisible to us.

The sun produces three types of ultraviolet light, two of which , UVA and UVB, are relevant to our health. UVA is responsible for deep skin wrinkling and possibly the worst kind of skin cancer, melanoma. UVB is thought to be the cause of sunburn, cataracts, and basal cell carcinoma, the most common type of skin cancer. While harmful in excess, UVB is necessary for health and life. UVB is what reacts with cholesterol (another "bad guy" necessary for life) in our skin to produce vitamin D.

Vitamin D, the sunshine vitamin, is best known as being necessary for calcium metabolism. Most people with osteoarthritis and musculoskeletal pain are deficient in vitamin D, causing calcium is deposited in cartilage. Low vitamin D leads to many other ailments, including depression, infertility, poor tooth development, osteoporosis, PMS and thyroid problems.Vitamin D also helps prevent colon, breast, and prostate cancers. It strengthens the immune system, preventing the flu, other infections, and autoimmune disorders.

According to the Institute of Medicine you can get adequate vitamin D by exposing your face and hands to the sun for twenty to thirty minutes, which will produce about 600 iu of vitamin D. In the winter most people will need a supplement. Some vitamin D is included in multivitamins, some calcium supplements, and cod liver oil. Most doctors now recommend at least 1000 iu per day.

Recent research suggests that the physiological requirement for adults may actually be much higher, in the range of 4000 to 5000 iu per day. Deficiency or overdose can be monitored by getting a serum 25(OH)D level and a calcium level.

Our human ancestors evolved near the equator, their naked skin exposed to the sun's UV-B, producing vastly more vitamin D than most modern lifestyles allow. Every organ in the body has vitamin D receptors, meaning the whole body needs the optimum amount to function correctly, and few people are getting enough.

Winter SADness

Many people find that they slow down, sleep more, stay indoors and feel like hibernating when the days get short and cold. About twenty percent of the US population, three quarters of whom are women, suffer from what is called seasonal affective disorder (SAD), with symptoms like depression, fatigue, carbohydrate craving, weight gain, and oversleeping. It is now known that this is caused by lack of light and can be treated by exposure to bright light for several hours a day.   Ordinary room light is not bright enough. You need a light source of ten thousand lux. Special lights are now available for this purpose. Light therapy is most effective when used in the morning. The bright light resets the body's biological clock, which may sometimes get out of phase with natural cycles of day and night.

Light stimulates synthesis of serotonin in the retina and brain, and stops production of melatonin. Melatonin is made in the pineal gland only in darkness, and is the body's natural sleep inducer. On short, dark winter days there may not be enough light to produce enough serotonin or to stop excess melatonin production. Depression can be caused by lack of serotonin or too much melatonin. The light treatment for SAD usually works in three to five days, faster, cheaper and without the side effects of antidepressants. Many people may benefit by getting outdoors and taking a walk in the morning sunlight, without glasses or sunglasses. This will also provide the benefit of exercise, another natural antidepressant.

According to Jacob Liberman, light not only affects our bodies directly, but also indirectly, through the foods we eat. Food can be thought of as light in solid form. All energy ultimately comes from sunlight, converted by chlorophyll in plants into chemical energy stored in food. Dr. Gabriel Cousins, author of _Spiritual Nutrition and the Rainbow Diet_, believes that nature has color-coded all foods, and that the color of a food correlates with the chakra of the same color, and helps to energize, balance and heal the glands, organs and nerve centers associated with that chakra. Dr. Cousins recommends a rainbow diet of live, colorful, full-spectrum foods to nourish the entire being. As I discussed earlier, antioxidants come in every color of the rainbow, including red lycopene, orange carotene, yellow lutein, green chlorophyll, blue anthocyanin, and purple resveratrol. We should avoid colorless white food (sugar, flour, rice) and eat a rainbow every day!

Chapter 28

Weather, Cycles and Health, Our Cosmic Connection

According to Pat Thomas, <u>Under the Weather</u>, one in three of us are "weather sensitive", women more than men, children more than adults. The new science of "Biometeorology" looks at the relationship between atmospheric and climate patterns around the world, and global health patterns. Whether we are aware of it or not, our reactions to weather show that our bodies interact with the natural environment at a very deep level.

We respond to weather at a biochemical level. Our skin, nose, lungs and muscles respond to the weight of the atmosphere, and the friction of the wind on our skin. Our joints may be sensitive to barometric pressure, allowing us to predict rain, by "feeling it in our bones".

The sun, (light and heat), water, wind and geomagnetic forces that make up weather are natural influences that define our life and evolution. In fact, these four elements, sun, water, air and earth, without which life cannot exist, were considered sacred, and worshiped and honored by many ancient societies. Each of these elements also has its destructive side: heat waves, floods, hurricanes, and desertification. Global warming, caused or aggravated by human activity, increases the severity of all these weather extremes.

The sun, along with the rotation of the earth, is responsible for one of the most important cycles in nature, for all plant and animal life, the diurnal or day/night cycle. Processes that take place in close to a twenty-four hour cycle are known as *circadian*, from Latin *circa dia*, "about a day". The sleep/wake cycle is the most obvious example. At regular intervals that may vary somewhat among individuals, the body becomes hungry, energized, tired, alert, or drowsy. Hormones such as cortisol, TSH and growth hormone rise and fall in predictable daily patterns governed partly by the light/dark cycle.

Timing of Drugs

Many arthritic diseases show a circadian pattern. Rheumatoid arthritis sufferers have more swelling and stiffness in the morning, while the pain of osteoarthritis, the wear and tear joint disorder that increases with time and age, is worse in the evening and at night. The time of day when a remedy or drug is taken affects its effectiveness and the incidence of side effects. Studies show that NSAIDS (non-steroidal anti-inflammatory drugs) cause much less damage to the stomach lining when taken at night rather than in the morning.

According to Pat Thomas, aerobic exercise is of most benefit between 4 and 7 pm, when our heart and lungs are stronger and our metabolic rate is highest. However, I don't believe this applies to everyone, because certain homeopathic types, like *Lycopodium, Sepia* and *Carcinosin*, are at their lowest energetic point at this time of day.

Jet Lag

Traveling across time zones can cause desynchronisation of our internal clocks with the light/dark cycle at our destination, known as jet lag. This is worse when flying east. Most people have a circadian pattern a little longer than 24 hours, making it easier to stay up later than to go to bed earlier. It normally takes one day to recover from each time zone crossed. This disruption can be eased by taking melatonin if you need to sleep earlier than your body clock tells you, or caffeine such as green or black tea or coffee if you need to delay your sleep time.

Moon Cycles

The monthly cycle corresponding to the phases of the moon is known as the circa lunar cycle. In primitive times before artificial lighting, women's cycles probably followed the phases of the moon, ovulating around the full moon, (the most romantic time for conception), and bleeding during the dark time. A study of one-hundred-forty-thousand live births in New York City in 1968 showed that fertility peaked at the third quarter phase of the moon. The researchers speculated that ovulation may be triggered by the decreasing level of illumination right after the full moon.

Chapter 29

Climate Truth

Al Gore's movie <u>An Inconvenient Truth</u> opened about a year after hurricane Katrina hit New Orleans. Before that disastrous event, I never heard mention of global warming or climate change on television. Even after that, it was rarely mentioned on commercial television, but there had been some documentaries on the topic on the Free Speech TV network.

There is a problem with the name. "Global warming" sounds like something nice. Who doesn't want to be warm and cozy? And aren't we all trying to go global these days. The previous terminology, "the greenhouse effect" was even worse; a place to grow beautiful plants, no matter what the weather. "Climate change" is too neutral; it doesn't imply that it's a bad thing. "Climate Crisis" is a better name. The president who lost the popular vote to Al Gore in 2000 (George W Bush) advised us not to quibble about whether global warming, which he wasn't sure existed, was man-made or a natural phenomenon. Climate Scientists now all agree that global warming is upon us, and most of it is caused by carbon dioxide produced by burning fossil fuels to run cars and power plants. Oil corporations make money when people burn more oil. Everyone running the country before 2008 seemed to be an oil man or woman, and our foreign policy was what you would expect if oil executives were running it.

The world-wide health effects of climate change have already begun. Mosquito-borne diseases like malaria are increasing, as tropical vectors spread into previously temperate zones. Food supplies are being affected, causing food riots in many areas. More violent weather is causing increased erosion of topsoil. Many plants and trees may not have the period of freezing winter cold needed before they can begin their spring blooming. Increased temperature adds to the harmful effects of insecticides causing the disappearance of honey bees which pollinate most of our fruits and vegetables.   More destructive hurricanes and tornadoes are destroying people, homes and farmland. Rising sea levels caused by melting glaciers are inundating island nations, and beginning to invade coastal cities, farmlands, and the sensitive ecological systems of tidal bays and estuaries, which are the nurseries for most fish and sea life.

As weather and rainfall patterns change, tropical areas like Africa are seeing deserts spread and starvation increase. Malnutrition affects the immune system, making people more susceptible to diseases like AIDS and malaria. Heat waves around the world are becoming more severe, causing more people to suffer heat stress, heart attacks and strokes.

SUV's in China?

Developing countries like India and China where people used to be too poor to think of buying cars, now want what we in the West have taken for granted. What if everyone in China drove an SUV?   Nobody, not even Americans, wants American gas guzzlers anymore. Detroit started getting into trouble when gas went to three dollars a gallon. There are long waiting lists for hybrids. China is leapfrogging over obsolete American internal combustion technology and developing more environmentally friendly vehicles, like electric cars. Unfortunately, however, the electricity to power those cars in China is being produced by burning coal. China is building a new coal-burning power plant every week!

Brazil has led the way by powering vehicles with fuel made from sugarcane, making them totally energy independent by the end of 2006. Some people in the US have converted diesel cars to run on used french fry oil from fast food places. Better to drive it than eat it!

Economic Collapse

Teddy Goldsmith, the editor of <u>The Ecologist</u> and founder of the Green Party in England, said years ago that the only thing that would stop global warming would be a worldwide economic collapse, as destructive as that would be. This collapse is now well under way and will be aggravated by massive economic losses caused by destructive weather events, and wars over dwindling resources like oil, food and water. The world may have already hit "peak oil", when the oil production from oil fields begins to decrease. This already happened in the US in the 1970's, and is happening now in Saudi Arabia.

Toxic Seafood

It is said that America has enough coal to power us for a hundred years, but this is no solution. Coal is the dirtiest fuel in existence, and there is no way to make it clean. Most of our electricity is generated by burning coal in power plants. Besides being a major source of greenhouse gases and acid rain, coal releases toxic heavy metals like mercury, arsenic, and lead into the environment. The toxins are in the smoke released high into the air by smokestacks, and fall with rain on land and sea. They are absorbed by plankton that form the diet of small fish, which are eaten by bigger fish, and accumulate in the food chain until big predators like tuna and swordfish are too toxic to eat.

In an attempt to decrease the release of carbon and heavy metals, scrubbers have been installed on smokestacks to collect the fly ash from burned coal, which is then stored in retention ponds. In December 2008, in one of these ponds used by one of fourteen coal-burning power plants owned by the Tennessee Valley Authority, a retention wall gave way, spilling coal ash sludge over two hundred to four hundred acres of land drained by the Emory River, a tributary of the Tennessee River, contaminating the source of water for millions of people downstream.

No Clean Coal

According to Matt Landon of United Mountain Defense, there is no such thing as clean coal. Coal is "dirty, dangerous and destructive from cradle to grave". The "cradle", surface mining, is extremely destructive to the environment. Whole mountain tops are removed by huge machines and dumped into valleys, destroying ecology and wildlife, and polluting streams and rivers. The "grave", when coal is burned, releases heavy metals and carbon dioxide. There is no way to make coal safe to mine or burn. Money being spent to create mythical "clean coal" would be better spent developing truly clean energy sources, solar and wind. During World War Two, auto plants were converted to produce tanks and warplanes. Now they should be converted to put laid-off auto workers back to work to produce solar devices, wind turbines and electric cars. Electric cars were made by General Motors in California in the 1990's, and worked perfectly well until they were all recalled and crushed.

American ingenuity should be put to work creating the new renewable energy economy for the world. Alternative energy sources like solar and wind are becoming cheaper and more available, and this process should be accelerated. Oil, gas and coal subsidies should be stopped and replaced by solar and wind subsidies and tax rebates. These are win-win solutions which will reduce our dependence of fossil fuels, decrease air pollution and global warming, and protect pristine areas like Alaska from more oil drilling. Let's hope it's not too late.

Chapter 30

No Nukes Now

Fossil fuels -- oil, gas and coal -- were laid down as excess plant and animal remains that built up over millions of years during the Age of Dinosaurs, the Triassic, Jurassic, and Cretaceous periods, the Carboniferous Era. Fossil fuels are the stored up energy of sunlight from eons ago. We are now burning up the "last hours of ancient sunlight". As fossil fuel supplies dwindle, is nuclear power the answer to our energy needs?

The first commercial nuclear power plant came on line in 1957, over sixty years ago. No new nuclear power plants have been built since the Three Mile Island meltdown in 1979. After fifty years of failure, Wall Street will not invest in them. No private insurance company will insure them. If new nuclear construction begins in the US, taxpayers will foot the bill.

Hiroshima to Fukushima

Scientific experts believe Japan's nuclear disaster to be far worse than governments are revealing to the public. "Fukushima is the biggest industrial catastrophe in the history of mankind," according to Arnold Gundersen, a former nuclear industry senior vice president. No nuclear reactors are designed to withstand an earthquake of magnitude 8.0. Yet there were eleven earthquakes greater than 8.5 last century, and there were already five in the first eleven years of the 21[st]century. Almost all were followed by tsunamis.

Even after Fukushima, Obama still endorsed nuclear power as a "clean energy" source, and wanted loan guarantees for corporations that build nuclear power plants. Obama claimed building more nukes would help prevent global warming. But what the nuclear industry and Obama did not admit was the fact that the overall nuclear "fuel cycle" - mining, milling, fuel fabrication, enrichment, and so on - contributes substantially to global warming.

In a nation-wide referendum here in Italy in June, 2011, ninety-five percent of voters said no to resuming our nuclear industry. All nuclear plants in Italy were closed down in 1987, after Chernobyl. The first solar power plant in Italy was built at Altomonte, in Cosenza, Calabria, a few dozen kilometers from where we live. It generates enough electricity to power 2800 households. Calabria is an ideal site for renewable energy. Most days are sunny, and there are frequent strong winds like the Scirocco from the south, and the Tramontana from the north.

Some so-called "environmentalists" think nukes are the answer to climate change. But after Three Mile Island, Chernobyl, Fukushima, and dozens of near-misses and radiation leaks, and the ever-mounting pile of nuclear waste that no one knows what to do with for the next hundred thousand years, people want no more of it, and have made their voices heard.

After massive protests by the Greens, Social Democrats, and tens of thousands of others, Germany decided to phase out all its nukes by 2022, and to continue its rapid deployment of renewables. Germany already has low per capita carbon dioxide emissions and plans to keep reducing it. The US, Canada and Australia have twice the emissions and seemingly no plan or intention of reforming.

Renewable power generation in Germany has increased substantially in the past twenty years. Germany has been called "the world's first major renewable energy economy". Renewable energy in Germany is mainly based on wind, solar and biomass. As of 2016, Germany had the world's third largest photovoltaic installed capacity, with 40 GW. Now that

Germany has the infrastructure in place, that percentage will climb rapidly, especially with the plummeting cost of photovoltaic solar. Germany and Italy are demonstrating to the world that we do not need dirty, dangerous nuclear power. Even France, which now gets most of its power from nukes, is investing heavily in renewables - far above minimum EU goals. If nukes were a better solution, France would be deploying more - but they're not.

Nuclear power is not the answer to climate change.

A nuclear power plant takes over ten years to construct and bring on line, during which time coal (the worst source of CO2) continues to be burnt unabated. And nukes are not "zero-carbon", as some claim.   Their lifecycle emissions are six times higher than wind and about double solar. Nukes also take resources away from low carbon renewables that can be rapidly deployed now. Nukes are more expensive than ever, while the cost of wind and solar continue to fall.

The majority of people in just about every country on the planet oppose nuclear power. Why can't the US have a referendum to determine if people want to be exposed to the catastrophic risks of nuclear power? People should have a say in how society is powered. Those who advocate one hundred percent renewables are on the right track - especially when entire countries like Germany and Italy are in agreement and committed to that policy.

Finally, all nuclear reactors create the raw materials for nuclear weapons, like plutonium, as a by-product. Attempting to reduce greenhouse-gas emissions through nuclear energy, thereby fueling the dangers of the ultimate global incendiary – nuclear war – could be the most tragic of all miscalculations.

Nuclear power is obsolete. It makes global warming worse, and diverts resources away from the true answer. The only solution to global climate change is renewable energy from solar, wind, geothermal, ocean thermal and tidal forces, and biofuels from plants that do not threaten and overprice the food supply, like perennial grasses, hemp, kudzu, algae, and certain trees and weeds. These green energy sources, along with increased efficiency and conservation, are our only hope for the future.

Clean Energy Jobs

We need to restructure taxes to remove subsidies on fossil fuels and subsidize green energy instead. We could have a Manhattan project to develop solar power, and reopen closed factories to produce efficient solar panels and photovoltaic roof tiles for every roof, and wind turbines for every backyard or village. We could revitalize our economy by producing clean energy for the world. Rooftop solar water heaters are spreading fast in Europe and China. The most promising energy source for the future is the almost limitless power of the sun.   Only a few percent of the world's deserts could collect enough solar energy to supply all energy needs for the world.

One of the easiest and most economical things you can do at home to reduce fossil fuel use and carbon dioxide production is to replace all incandescent light bulbs with compact fluorescent bulbs that use only one forth as much electricity and last years longer. I did this in my own house (in New Jersey) twenty years ago and only had to replace one since then. Even though these bulbs contain mercury, (and should be disposed of properly), they save so much electricity, which means less mercury pollution produced by coal-burning power plants, that the overall environmental mercury burden is reduced. Compact fluorescents have now been replaced by LEDs, Light Emitting Diodes, which avoid the mercury problem, but may cause other health problems, due to excessive blue light. If everyone used energy efficient light bulbs, world electricity use could be cut by twelve percent, according to <u>Plan B 3.0</u>, by Lester Brown, enough to close over seven hundred of the world's coal-fired power plants. Here in Italy, where I live now, everyone uses compact fluorescent light bulbs or LEDs.

Part 5

Future Evolution

Chapter 31

Seafood and Evolution

"The birds are coming. It's the end of the world!"   In the Hitchcock thriller, <u>The Birds</u>, the seagulls and other birds are organized into a conspiracy of revenge against humans who have exploited them since the beginning of time. Now we fear migrating birds not for their evil thoughts, but for diseases they carry, like avian flu, through no fault of their own. Why have birds suddenly become so susceptible to the flu virus, which has always been around in birds and never caused much trouble?

Migrating birds have been flying over the oceans, from pole to pole and across time zones before there were time zones.   Why have they suddenly started coming down with bird flu now? Is something compromising their immune systems? Is it something in their diet? Mostly they're flying over the ocean, so what do they have to eat along the way? There's nothing in the sea but seafood. What is in seafood that makes humans afraid to eat it now, in spite of its abundance of omega-3 essential fatty acids vitally needed by our brains and hearts?

Why Humans Walk Upright

The abundance of sea food in our diet as we evolved on tropical shores provided the EPA and DHA fuel that allowed our brains to expand and evolve. Wading out into shallow seas to catch fish and shellfish provided the most perfect incentive to adopt an upright posture; that is, keeping our heads above water! We perfected the art of swimming as infants, learning to swim before we could walk. Even today a newborn baby placed in water will automatically hold its breath and paddle.

We became the "naked ape" not because of fanciful theories about sexual attractiveness, but simply because, for swimmers, fur is a drag! Smooth skinned swimmers had a better chance to escape sharks, as well as getting away from tigers on shore. The Aquatic Ape theory of human evolution also explains the enigma of the fat baby. Compared to other primate infants, human babies are born round faced and chubby, in spite of the difficulty for the pregnant mother of getting enough extra calories to put fat on the baby, as well as the burden of carrying that heavy baby around once it's born. The only animals that benefit from a layer of body fat are those that spend a lot of time in water. Fat babies float! Sea mammals like dolphins and seals, as well as humans, but no other primates, have a subcutaneous fat layer that provides buoyancy, insulation and streamlining, needed for an aquatic lifestyle.

The Toxic Sea

Now, thanks to human industrial activities and burning of fossil fuel, the nourishing sea that gave us birth and allowed us to evolve, has become a toxic cesspool that may bring about our devolution and death. Coal-burning power plants spew mercury into the air, which falls in rain, flows into rivers and ends up in the sea. Tiny sea plants and animals absorb the mercury, which ends up in fish, eaten by migrating sea birds.

Mercury is toxic to the immune system and most body processes. Dolphins also live on fish, and they too have been succumbing in increasing numbers to mysterious viral illnesses. It seems likely to me that fish-eating birds and mammals are being immunocompromised by mercury and other heavy metals contaminating their food supply, not to mention pesticides used on farms and gardens that all eventually wash into the sea and end up in fatty tissues of sea creatures.

Chapter 32
Blood Type and Evolution

According to Peter D'Adamo, <u>Eat Right for Your Type,</u> people with Type O blood are descended from hunters. They need red meat and vigorous exercise to feel strong. They are the warriors. Native Americans are predominantly Type O. A warrior culture is not a warlike culture. American Indians say their warriors were the defenders of the tribe, not conquerors. The young men warriors were also the hunters. They treated the animals with respect, taking only what was needed for their own tribe's survival. The animals were as free as the hunters until their "good day to die". Surely the meat from these wild animals raised by nature must have had different effects on the human body than meat raised today in animal factories, fed grain and dead animals instead of the native grasses and plants that were their natural diet.

The nutritional content of meat from wild game animals, such as that consumed by native "First Peoples" all over the world, as well as our own Paleolithic ancestors, was very different from modern factory meat. It was actually closer in fatty acid content to seafood, wild fish, the food that allowed our human brain to develop millions of years ago. Grass-fed beef and free-range pastured chickens are now becoming more popular and available. They are much better for the health of consumers, and the earth.

The Inuit Enigma

In the 1950's it was marveled that Eskimos, as Inuit peoples were then called, were virtually free of cardiovascular disease, in spite of their high fat, mostly meat diet. (The word Eskimo means eater of raw meat.) But the fat in that diet was not the highly saturated fat produced by grain-fed pigs and cows. Bovines actually convert the polyunsaturated fats found in grasses into saturated storage fat, which was thought to clog your arteries.   The native peoples of Alaska lived mostly on fish, and sea animals that ate fish.   Their fat was the polyunsaturated type high in omega-3 essential fatty acids, EPA and DHA, needed for a healthy heart and brain.

Type A's

People with Type A blood are not hunters, but "gatherers" (they like to gather together). They like to live together in communities and work cooperatively, according to D'Adamo. The higher carbohydrate levels in the more vegetarian diet that benefits Type A's also tends to raise serotonin levels, which has a calming effect needed by Type A's.

Serotonin is made from the amino acid, tryptophan, but its production is favored by a high carbohydrate diet. Carbohydrate foods cause release of insulin which causes most amino acids to go out of the blood stream into the cells, except for tryptophan, which then has no competition crossing into the brain, where it is converted to serotonin. Therefore a vegetarian diet or a spaghetti dinner would tend to have a calming effect. People with type A blood, who, coincidentally, also tend to be the "Type A personality," benefit from things that calm them down, like vegetarian or high carbohydrate food, and quieting exercises like yoga, tai chi, and meditation.

Type A's multiplied during the Neolithic Age, ten thousand years ago, when humans began to invent agriculture. After the end of the last Ice Age, the earth became warmer and dryer, forests receded and grasslands expanded, (with more or less help from humans, as is still going on today.) Women gathered the seeds of the abundant grasses, wild ancestors of wheat, native to the Fertile Crescent. Also known as Mesopotamia, the land between (meso) the rivers (potamia), the Tigris and the Euphrates, this area has been called the "Cradle of Civilization".   Most of the cultivated plants and domesticated animals of Western Civilization had their origin in this area. This is also the site of the Biblical Garden of Eden, through which the Tigris and Euphrates rivers flowed, now known as Iraq.

The Agricultural Revolution

During the "agricultural revolution", ten thousand years ago, people whose digestive systems could begin to handle the carbohydrates and glutens in the seeds of grasses that eventually developed into wheat, oats, rye and barley, had an abundant new food source and were able to greatly expand their population. Their immune systems also changed so that they became able to thrive in much greater population density than that of nomadic hunter/gatherers. Infectious diseases carried by rodents that lived in the grain stores sometimes spread to humans. The survivors of the epidemics passed on their resistance to diseases that were more likely to spread in closer living conditions.

The Importance of Cats

Women, who were the first gardeners and growers of the grain that was the economic basis of the community, domesticated cats to protect the grain stores from rodents. Actually, cats may have domesticated themselves by hanging around areas where there were plenty of mice and warm sheltered areas, and friendly women and children who did not try to harm their kittens and actually protected them from predators.

By keeping the rodent population under control, cats helped prevent epidemic diseases like the bubonic plague, spread by fleas that live on rodents. The Fourteenth Century bubonic plague epidemic, known as the Black Death, killed a quarter of the population of Europe. One reason the plague may have spread so widely is because so many cats were killed along with their owners, women who were accused of witchcraft, tortured

194

and executed by the misogynistic patriarchal Inquisition, intent on wiping out the last vestiges of goddess worship and women's rites.

Neolithic people all over the world lived in agrarian egalitarian matrilineal communities, and worshiped the Great Mother represented by the cycles of nature and the moon. Women's monthly cycles were fashioned by the moon, by the effect of moonlight on women's hormonal cycles.

The hunting lifestyle, in which the human is at the top of the food chain, requires a lot of forest for the deer and rabbits, or prairie/savannah/steppes for the wild game herds to find enough vegetable matter to maintain their numbers.   Grasses, with their nutrient-dense seed heads, were becoming abundant in the grasslands that expanded as the forests decreased, (probably due to a combination of climate changes and human activity.)

Type A humans descended from ancestors who through a lucky genetic mutation developed enzymes that allowed them to exploit this abundant new resource, poorly tolerated by Type O hunters. Type O's, like western American Indian tribes, who attempt to live on a high grain diet, (especially the white man's refined white flour), are prone to develop diabetes, obesity and heart disease. Many have found that getting back to a more natural native diet helps prevent these diseases of "civilization".

Type B's

Type B people, according to D'Adamo's blood type theory, are natural leaders. They are descended from herders, shepherds, (leaders of sheep?) They tend to be benevolent caretakers, shepherds of society. Another lucky mutation allowed them to digest lactose, milk sugar, still indigestible to many people of other types. Lactose tolerance in Northern Europeans permitted northern (and inland) expansion by providing a vitamin D source (sheep, goat, and cow's milk) other than sunlight and fish.

"The biblical Hebrews were a nomadic pastoral and patriarchal people, tribes of sheepherders and warriors who invaded land belonging to the matriarchal Canaanites," according to <u>The Great Cosmic Mother</u> by Monica Sjoo and Barbara Mor.

Herders learned from raising their herds, the secrets of the male role in reproduction, unknown to men in earlier hunter/gatherer societies, but always known to women, as they saw that their bodies stopped bleeding in tune with the dark moon for ten moon cycles, while their body became rounder and rounder like the full moon, and then a new human being appeared. Women kept this secret from men for a long time, while they invented moon calendars to keep track of when babies were due, and when to plant and harvest garden crops.

Meat and Aggression?

Is there something in a high meat/milk diet that might contribute to a more male dominated, warlike, expansionist lifestyle? Could it be the higher cholesterol, source of hormones like cortisol, the adrenal stress hormone, and the male hormone testosterone (as well as female hormones estrogen and progesterone)? Meat also supplies more zinc, which is needed to produce testosterone. Protein supplies amino acids, especially tyrosine, the precursor of adrenalin, the hormone of thrills, stress, energy, and adrenalin highs from doing dangerous things. Tyrosine also produces norepinephrine, the neurotransmitter responsible for anger, assertion, and ego. A high meat diet supplies more catecholamines relative to indolamines (serotonin).   Animals chased and killed in a hunt may have really high adrenalin levels. Is any of this absorbed by the eater? Are meat eaters more aggressive?

They would probably have to be in order to be successful hunters.   Many people find that they feel more peaceful (or maybe too passive) on a vegetarian diet, because of higher levels of serotonin induced by a high carbohydrate plant-based diet.

Chapter 33
Evolution – Two Paths

My solar-powered watch keeps resetting itself. When it doesn't get enough light, it shuts down and starts over. I think it's suffering from nostalgia. It keeps setting itself back to Saturday, January 1st, 2000, before all the bad stuff started happening. The world had just survived Y2K. Planes hadn't fallen out of the sky. Banks didn't lose all records, as many had feared. It took thousands of software engineers working day and night to prevent TEOTWAWKI (the end of the world as we know it), when computers clicked over from '99 to 2000.

Twentieth Century computers were designed with only two digit spaces for the year. It was feared that when computers clicked over from '99 to '00, they would "think" it was time to start over and lose all their records. At midnight on New Years' Eve 2000, the world celebrated, knowing that civilization had not ended. It will take more than a technological fix to save us this time. As John Lennon said, "you've got to change your mind instead."

In the late Nineteenth Century, "by a bizarre legal alchemy," corporations gradually acquired the legal status of a human being (recently concretized by the Supreme Court in the "Citizens United" decision of 2010!) But if a corporation is a person, it is certainly not a normal person, but a sociopath, unaffected by normal human emotions. Its only purpose, by law, is to increase profits to shareholders, no matter the cost to society. Corporations today control everything, including most of the world's food supply. Shopping at your local food co-op or farmers' market is one way to get around the corporations, subverting the dominant paradigm (the dominance paradigm).

Carl Sagan (in <u>The Varieties of Scientific Experience</u>), and Rianne Eisler (in <u>The Chalice and the Blade)</u>, both describe two different models of human society:
1) Dominance hierarchies, where some people have power over others, for example, male over female, slave master over slave, factory owner over workers.
2) Egalitarian or partnership societies, as found in many indigenous peoples and pre-patriarchal societies.

Make Love, Not War

Even our nearest relatives, the chimpanzees and bonobos, represent the same bifurcation. Chimps have dominance hierarchies; males dominate females, and different groups have border skirmishes when territory is invaded. Bonobo society seems to be based on the principle of "make love, not war". These animals are highly sexual and use sex to settle all disputes. Everybody gets as much sex as they want. There is plenty of food and everyone shares. When two groups meet, instead of fighting, they have a party, and share the available food. They are vegetarian, eating leaves, shoots and buds of succulent plants.

Incidentally (or not), one food that may be included in their diet is the hemp (cannabis) plant. It is grown by the pygmies who inhabit the same area of the Congo as bonobos, "their only cultivated crop," according to Carl Sagan, in <u>The Dragons of Eden</u>. Hemp seed (available at health food stores, grown in Canada), is one of the most highly nutritious foods in the world. It has higher quality protein than soy, and contains all the essential fatty acids, including omega-3 and GLA. Populations have survived famines on nothing but hemp seed.

Animals, even cats, have been known to eat growing hemp plants and hemp seeds. It would be surprising if bonobos did not include this highly nutritious plant in their diet. Maybe that's what gives them their peaceful personality.

Historical and evolutionary evidence indicates that both pathways are available to human nature: the dominator model, or the partnership paradigm. Let us all strive to steer society in the direction of cooperation. And remember, helping and sharing raise serotonin levels in both helper and helped, preventing depression and producing a joyful "Helper's High".

Chapter 34

Helper's High and Winner's High

The cover article in the premier issue of <u>Scientific American MIND</u>, "The Samaritan Paradox," tries to explain how the phenomenon of the kindness of strangers could have come about. In a "dog eat dog world", how could altruism have evolved? First of all, dogs don't eat dogs. Dogs, and their ancestors the wolves, cooperate in the hunt to catch food for the group. Many animals exhibit forms of altruism toward kin, particularly the care of mothers for offspring. If an animal mother did not take care of her babies, they would not survive, and genes for this aberrant behavior would not be passed on.

According to the <u>MIND</u> article, *Homo sapiens* is the only species capable of strong altruism even toward people they are not related to. (Of course, we are also the only species capable of genocide.) But helping others without expectation of personal benefit seems to contradict the struggle for survival. Charles Darwin's 1859 treatise <u>The Origin of Species</u> described the survival of the fittest in the struggle for food and reproduction. Less well known is his 1874 writing, in <u>The Descent of Man</u>, that a tribe whose members cooperated with each other "would be victorious over most other tribes, and this would be natural selection."

Helper's High

One reason for the evolution of altruism is that helping others has a natural antidepressant effect and promotes a feeling of well-being. People help each other because it feels good. The sense of well-being one experiences from helping or giving has been called a "Helper's High". This effect is thought to be mediated by serotonin, or possibly by oxytocin, the same hormone involved in giving birth and lactation.

In fact, it has been discovered that the act of helping actually raises one's serotonin level. Serotonin is the neurotransmitter responsible for feelings of contentment and satisfaction. Serotonin is released in the brain by sharing, cooperative activities, communication, and collaboration. Depression is thought to be due to lack of serotonin, and is usually treated by SSRIs, antidepressants that raise serotonin. It is an amazing discovery that serotonin can be raised simply by helping!

Helping actually raises the serotonin level in <u>both</u> the helper and the helped, according to Wayne Dyer, author of many self help books. This may explain the significance of the biblical proverb that it is more blessed to give than to receive, since giving raises the serotonin level in both parties. If this fact became widely known, it could start a new, healthy chain reaction of behavior change that would benefit everyone! (Except pharmaceutical companies that make antidepressants.) Serotonin levels go up not only in the helper and the one who is helped, but even in people who observe this activity. (That's why "feel good" movies make you feel good.)

According to John Gray, author of <u>Men Are from Mars, Women Are From Venus</u>, ninety percent of those who seek counseling for depression are women. Women derive great benefit from counseling or talk therapy or just talking to a friend. Women tend to have much lower brain serotonin levels than men, and need sharing and talking with other people to get their serotonin up. (Otherwise they may crave carbohydrates as another, biochemical, way of getting it up.)

Women are more likely than men to respond to serotonin-raising drugs or supplementing with serotonin precursors like tryptophan and 5-hydroxy tryptophan (5HTP). According to Wayne Dyer, women should not depend on men for the amount of talking and sharing they require to supply their serotonin needs. Men usually have plenty of serotonin. Men are looking for ways to raise a different neurotransmitter, dopamine.

Winner's High

Men suffering from depression are likely to be low in dopamine. Rather than anxiety and agitation, low dopamine depression is characterized by lethargy, boredom, and lack of drive. Dopamine levels can be raised by things like competition, sports, challenges, risk-taking, winning, being right, solving problems, making connections, completing circuits, and task oriented behavior. Some depressed males, especially young men and teenage boys, tend to have very low dopamine levels, and self-medicate by seeking out danger and life-threatening behavior. Dopamine is a precursor of adrenalin - which makes them feel alive. People with low dopamine, mostly men, but also some women, need and seek out competition, confrontation, or task-oriented work to stimulate dopamine production and sustain dopamine levels.

Winning obviously has survival value. So does being right, being able to predict what will happen. Both are rewarded by a shot in the brain of dopamine, what I call a "Winner's High", probably one of the brain's most ancient reward systems. The dopamine high is addictive. You miss it when it goes, resulting in craving, depression, the low that follows a manic high, whether natural or self-induced.

Probably even vicariously watching someone win releases the dopamine reward, which would explain why you feel so good when your team wins, and why many men seem to be so dependent on, even addicted to, spectator sports.

Dopamine is made in the brain from tyrosine or phenylalanine, amino acids that can be useful as part of a treatment program for depression or drug withdrawal. Children with ADD and ADHD, ninety percent of whom are boys, also have very low dopamine levels, according to John Gray.

Their disruptive, hyperactive behavior is a way of getting their dopamine levels up, so they feel better.

Chapter 35

Art and Science, Heart and Silence of Breath

The Art

The art of breathing goes along with the practice of meditation, concentration on the breath to exclude the mind's mostly frivolous verbal chatter about the past or future, and focus on how the body is breathing, <u>now</u>. Breathing is what the body does naturally and unconsciously, but unlike other automatic functions, it can also come under conscious control. Becoming aware of the breath is one way the mind can learn to consciously control itself. Three long, slow breaths can release the body/mind into the "alpha" state in which both hemispheres work together.

"Meditation is a mental state that insulates against stress," according to Jose Silva, who developed a simple method of meditation, relaxation, and visualization to regain and maintain mental and physical health. The Silva method has been taught to millions of people in over eighty countries since 1966. His forty-day self-training program, described in his 1989 book, <u>You the Healer</u>, begins with counting backward from one hundred to one, while in a relaxed seated position with eyes closed. Silva discovered that counting backward is a simple, effective way to slow brainwaves from the fast, active, working, narrow focus, high stress "beta" state, to the relaxed, middle range alpha state, between waking and light sleep, "the center of the brainwave frequency spectrum, where mind and awareness become attuned to the right brain hemisphere."

After a few weeks of practice, one is able to enter the alpha state at will by simply taking three deep breaths while mentally saying or visualizing the number "three", three times on the first exhalation, the number "two", three times on the second exhalation, and the number "one", three times on the third exhalation. In alpha the mind can instruct the body, "I will always maintain a perfectly healthy body and mind," while visualizing healing taking place in one's body.

The Science

Deepening the breath increases intake of oxygen. Slowing the breath increases retention of carbon dioxide (CO_2). Isn't that a bad thing? Not necessarily. People who breathe too fast, or hyperventilate from excitement, lose too much CO_2, which changes the pH (acidity) of their blood. This affects the solution of ions like calcium and magnesium, causing numbness, tingling and anxiety. The cure is simple. Breathing into a paper bag normalizes CO_2 and pH level, and restores calm. The higher carbon dioxide level produced by slow meditative breathing increases blood flow through the right middle cerebral artery of the brain, activating the right hemisphere.

Ever since humans began to read and write, according to Leonard Schlain, in <u>The Alphabet versus the Goddess</u>, our brains have been unbalanced. The left hemisphere contains the speech centers and controls the right hand, the one that writes, in most of us. The "dominant" left brain performs linear, sequential, digital, and time oriented functions. The right hemisphere is thought to be non-linear, timeless, analog, and oriented to spatial relations. Art, music, and appreciation of nature are thought to reside there. Meditative breathing induces a state of relaxation, and increased activity of the right brain. The overworked left brain rests from narrowly focused concentration, the "fight or flight", high stress state frequently needed for survival, but aging the body too quickly if it can't be turned off.

Researchers working with biofeedback equipment have found that in the fast wave beta state the brainwaves pulsate at fourteen to twenty-one Hertz. In alpha the brainwaves slow to eight to thirteen Hz, on their way down to theta, light sleep, at four to seven Hz, and finally deep sleep at less than four Hz. Biofeedback research scientists have discovered that at the alpha level, people become able to control body functions previously thought to be automatic and not under conscious control, like blood pressure, pulse rate, temperature of hands and feet, relief from headaches and tension related pain, and accelerated healing of the body.

Neuropsychologist Les Fehmi, Ph D, director of the Princeton Biofeedback Centre, with whom I worked for many years, was one of the first scientists to discover that skilled meditators in the alpha state experience "synchronous rhythm", when brainwaves from both hemispheres move together in phase, with the same amplitude and frequency. This state is associated with moments of peak lucidity, intuition and heightened awareness. Dr.Fehmi developed a technique he calls "Open Focus" to teach people to enter the alpha state by imagining "empty space" sequentially in all areas of the mind and body, described in his 2007 book, The Open Focus Brain, and his 2010 book, Dissolving Pain.

The Heart

According to Paul Pearsall PhD, in his 2000 book Wishing Well, new research supports what he has always espoused throughout his many books, that the heart is not just a pump, but an organ that thinks, feels, and communicates our "heartfelt intentions." The heart is the body's strongest producer of electromagnetic energy, forty times more powerful than the brain. Its energy can be measured almost twenty feet from the body. The heart represents the unconscious mind, in poetry and ancient texts: "as a man thinketh in his heart, so is he". According to Candace Pert, in Molecules of Emotion, "the body is the unconscious mind!" The unconscious mind may also be the non-verbal right hemisphere, perhaps still connected to the ancient wisdom of humans before the development of speech.

The Silence

Silence is something rarely experienced these days. With constant verbal bombardment by television, radio, cell phones, talking, reading, when does the brain get a chance to think? Or stop thinking and feel? People are busy solving immediate problems and have no time to think about what is happening in the world, or even in their own bodies. Turn everything off, take three deep breaths in silence, and give your brain a mini-vacation.

Afterword
Natural vs Synthetic, Herb vs Drug

What is Natural Medicine? Natural Medicine refers to treatment of medical conditions by means of substances and modalities that occur in nature, such as whole foods and nutritional supplements. Supplements are concentrated sources of nutrients such as vitamins, minerals, and fatty acids which occur naturally in foods. Herbs or botanical remedies are also part of Natural Medicine. They are plants or plant parts such as the flower, leaf or root, which are used, fresh or dried, in their whole form, containing a myriad of different substances which all work together and work with the body to promote gentle healing. Different components may have antagonistic or complimentary effects which modify or smooth out the main effect.

A drug, on the other hand, is a single chemical compound, often extracted, as the so-called "active ingredient", from a plant or other natural source, such as digitalis from Foxglove (Digitalis purpurea) leaf. The herbal preparation of digitalis leaf gave warning signs of impending overdose or toxicity, such as digestive upsets, so it could be decreased or stopped before dangerous cardiac arrhythmias occurred. With digitalis in the pure drug form, life-threatening abnormal heart rhythms can come on suddenly without warning if the dosage is not carefully monitored.

After a single substance is extracted from a plant or synthesized in a laboratory, it is then usually chemically modified in some way, such as adding extra molecular groups, to make it slightly different from the original source, so that it can be patented as a drug. (No matter if the patented modified substance is more toxic or harder for the body to metabolize than the original form.)

One reason that conventional allopathic doctors prefer to use synthetic drugs and non-bioidentical hormones is that their medical school education, subsidized by pharmaceutical companies, is biased in favor of treating with pharmaceutical drugs, while denigrating or ignoring the use of botanical, nutritional and homeopathic remedies. It is ironic that medical doctors refer to themselves as allopaths, without realizing that this derisive term was coined by Hahnemann to distinguish the "old school" physicians who gave drugs that cause "other suffering" ("allo" is Greek for other, "pathos" for suffering) from homeopaths!

Sugar is an Addictive Drug

By the scientific definitions described above, white sugar is a drug, a single chemical compound extracted from a whole plant such as sugar cane which contains all the nutrients and fiber needed to metabolize the sugar contained in it in a healthy way. Refined white sugar contains no nutrients and actually depletes the body of the vitamins and minerals needed to break it down. It is one of the most addictive drugs.

Cocaine, of course, is another pure, white, addictive drug extracted from a plant, which causes severe environmental destruction to the South American rain forest, as it devastates its consumers. The leaf of the coca plant (Erythroxylon coca) in its whole natural form has been chewed by the Indians of the Peruvian Andes for thousands of years.   The leaves are highly nutritious, full of vitamins and minerals which allow the Indians to benefit harmlessly from the small amount of cocaine contained in them, which, indeed, is what allows them to survive the low oxygen levels at such high altitudes. In fact, homeopathic coca leaf is used as a treatment for altitude sickness.

On the other hand, marijuana is obviously not a drug, but a nonaddictive herb, the leaves and flowers of the Cannabis sativa plant, used in the whole natural form, smoked or eaten. It has many medicinal uses, such as treatment of glaucoma, muscle spasticity as in multiple sclerosis, epilepsy in children, nausea from chemotherapy, and even many types of cancer. It also helps prevent lung cancer in tobacco smokers. In Europe, most cannabis smokers mix it with tobacco. They think it strange that Americans smoke their marijuana plain.   As of this writing, marijuana may be legally used for medicinal purposes with a doctor's prescription in most states of the US.   The erroneous classification of cannabis as a "narcotic" drug dates back to 1937, when the cannabis plant, also known as hemp, was first made illegal, the same year nylon, the first synthetic fiber, was patented by DuPont. (Coincidence?)

Before 1937, everything that is now made out of nylon or plastic was made out of hemp, the strongest natural fiber in the world. An article in "Popular Mechanics", published in February, 1938, (prepared for publication in the spring of 1937, just before hemp was outlawed), forecast that it would be a billion dollar crop, in 1938! This was because a machine called a hemp decorticator had just been invented, which would have made it much easier to separate the strong hemp fibers from the pith, or "hurds" of the stalk. The hurds would also have had numerous uses, including making paper, instead of using trees. If hemp had not been outlawed, the world would be in a much less polluted state today. The hurds could have been used to make biodegradeable forms of plastic which could have competed on a level playing field with the petrochemical synthetics that will remain and degrade the earth and seas forever.

This is one of the earliest instances of replacing something natural, which fits into the cycles of nature, with synthetics, man-made products of coal and oil, that never existed in nature, that nature's microorganisms cannot break down. Synthetics like plastic bags and bottles that are thoughtlessly used once and thrown away end up in the oceans where they accumulate forever, poisoning and choking aquatic life. Discarded nylon fishing nets remain in the sea, trapping and killing fish and other sea creatures in perpetuity. There are large areas in all the oceans permanently filled with floating bits of plastic. Many sea animals eat them and die. They mistake floating plastic bags for edible jellyfish. (I am happy to report that, as of January 2011, Italy is the first country in Europe to outlaw production of nonbiodegradable plastic bags!) Pesticide residues, washed by rain from farms and lawns, end up in the sea, along with thousands of other toxic chemicals that are sickening sea creatures, from the algae that produce most of the earth's oxygen, to the whales and dolphins.

The End of Evolution?

If ocean life is killed off, can humanity survive? Will we be able to maintain our human intelligence and forward evolution which was fueled by seafood, the only source of omega-3 EPA and DHA, one of the main structural lipids of the human brain?   Will future generations look back on the Golden Age of the Twentieth Century, when people were intelligent enough to create all those wonders, thanks to the brain-food that used to fill the seas?

Synthetic drugs excreted unchanged in human waste also accumulate in waterways, along with pesticide runoff from farms and lawns, harming fish and wildlife. Natural herbs and homeopathic remedies leave no toxic residue, and organic, locally grown food promotes healthy human beings and a healthy environment.

Appendix

Biotypes of Alcoholism

I presented the following paper, dealing with nutrition and alcoholism, over thirty-five years ago, on April 4th, 1982, at the National Council on Alcoholism meeting in Washington DC, while I was working at the Princeton Brain Bio Center. Dorothy Mullen, who researched this topic recently in preparation for founding Suppers for Sobriety, came up with pretty much the same information. In other words, apparently, little research has been done on nutrition and alcoholism in the last 35 years.

Alcoholism is a physiological addiction that may develop in about ten percent of alcohol drinkers. Studies since the turn of the Twentieth Century have shown that the tendency to alcoholism often runs in families. Many studies on adopted children, twins, and half-siblings show that there is a genetic tendency to alcoholism, rather than just an abnormal behavior learned by imitation of parents.

How does this inherited tendency produce alcoholism, and can anything be done to modify it? According to Roger Williams, the eminent biochemist who discovered the vitamin pantothenic acid (B5), the genetic tendency to alcoholism can be overcome by good nutrition. Dr. Williams, who published his book <u>Prevention of Alcoholism through Nutrition </u>in 1951, expressed the belief that no one who followed good nutritional practices would ever become an alcoholic.

Experiments done in Dr. Williams' lab show that animals which normally would never drink alcohol can be induced to choose alcohol solutions in preference to water, after being fed a diet high in sugar, or a diet deficient in certain nutrients. When a completely adequate diet is restored, the animals will no longer drink alcohol.

Dr. Williams' experiments sought to answer the question of why certain individuals become alcoholic and others don't. He chose rats as an experimental animal to demonstrate individual differences. Twenty rats were put in separate cages and given a choice of water or 10% alcohol.

The individual rats had very different patterns of behavior. Some drank very little alcohol at any time; some drank a little at first, and then gradually increased. Some drank heavily right from the beginning. Some drank at periodic intervals separated by a few days of abstinence. After several years of investigations, Dr. Williams had some understanding of why individual animals behaved so differently, and why some chose to drink and others did not. He found inborn or hereditary differences in the metabolism of different animals, even though they were from the same inbred strain. Humans would have much wider variation.

He found that the animals that did not drink alcohol were receiving everything that they, as individuals, needed from their diet. Rats that chose alcohol were found to have some nutritional deficiency, because they had an inborn higher requirement for a certain particular element. Experiments were done omitting one particular vitamin from the diet of a rat; this resulted in heavy drinking. But when the vitamin was restored, drinking dropped suddenly, often in one day, to a very low level.

This experiment was repeated for vitamin A, thiamine (B1), riboflavin (B2), pantothenic acid (B5), and pyridoxine (B6). A deficiency of any one of these vitamins caused increased alcohol intake, which returned to normal when the missing vitamin was supplied. These experiments firmly established the close relationship between diet and the biological urge to drink.

Other experiments done by doctors at Loma Linda University in California showed similar results. Rats on a "typical teenage diet", high in refined carbohydrates and marginally low in vitamins and minerals, drank five times as much alcohol as rats on a balanced diet. When the equivalent of eighteen cups of coffee was added, alcohol intake increased by thirteen percent. When vitamins and minerals were added, there was a significant decrease in alcohol intake.

Dr. Williams' studies over a sixty year period show that every person has a distinctive metabolism and a unique pattern of nutritional needs. Requirements for specific nutrients may vary by five-fold or more. Some people are more vulnerable to alcoholism because they have greater requirements for nutrients involved in the metabolism of alcohol. When these individuals get inadequate nutrition (which always accompanies heavy drinking), some of their deficiencies become so severe that appetite-controlling mechanisms in the brain become deranged and no longer demand nourishing food, desiring only alcohol.

To prevent alcoholism or help alcoholics recover, Dr. Williams recommended education of alcoholics to eat nutritionally superior foods, and avoid not only alcohol, but also sugar and all refined foods. He recommended high potency nutritional supplements emphasizing B vitamins, zinc, and magnesium, known to be deficient in alcoholics, and also special supplements such as l-glutamine, which reduces alcohol as well as sugar craving.

A drinking alcoholic derives a large portion of his caloric intake from alcohol, which supplies only calories, no protein, vitamins or minerals. The average alcoholic consumes 120 - 140 grams (4 -5 ounces) of alcohol per day, supplying about 1200 calories, half or more of the daily requirement. Even if the other half of the diet were excellent, which is unlikely, the alcoholic would not be able to meet protein vitamin and mineral needs.

In addition, alcohol interferes with the absorption of several nutrients, including B1, B12, and folic acid. Over half of alcoholics have intestinal damage, or deficiency of the pancreatic enzymes needed to digest fats, essential fatty acids, fat soluble vitamins A, D, and E, and protein. In addition, liver damage impairs conversion of vitamins to their active forms.

Deficiency of magnesium and B1 may be responsible for hangover symptoms, insomnia, and withdrawal symptoms such as tremors or shakes. Zinc deficiency causes low testosterone levels, with impotence and atrophy of male sex organs. This will often be restored to normal after several months of abstinence, and is a great incentive for some patients. Zinc is also required for conversion of vitamin A to the active form, retinol, in the eye. Night blindness results from deficiency of zinc or vitamin A, both lacking in alcoholics. Night blindness in alcoholics probably contributes to their high rate of highway crashes, since most alcohol-related crashes occur at night, even though there is less traffic then. With impaired night vision and delayed adaptation to darkness, a driver is blinded for a much longer time by the headlights of a passing car.

Some of the earliest practical work in treatment of alcoholism with nutrition was done by Doctors Humphrey Osmond and Abram Hoffer in Canada, who had pioneered the treatment of schizophrenia with massive doses of niacin and vitamin C, in the early 1950's. Realizing that alcoholism could produce behavioral and perceptual changes resembling psychosis, they tried the same treatment on alcoholics. Hoffer and Osmond cooperated with Bill W, cofounder of AA, to develop nutritional guidelines to go along with the spiritual guidance and psychological support provided by AA. Vitamins have been donated to AA by manufacturers and have been used for years as part of the treatment of many alcoholics.

A study on massive doses of niacin in treatment of alcoholism was started by Russell Smith in Michigan in1966, on 507 alcoholics. All were previous long-time treatment failures who had been in state mental hospitals, private psychotherapy, legal punitive therapy and AA. They were treated with 4000 mg or more of niacin daily, along with vitamin C, 500 mg twice a day. Of fifty-seven percent who could be reached for follow-up at the end of five years, and had continued on the treatment, forty-two percent had excellent results, with total abstinence for two or more years, emotional stability, and normal psychological state. Not a single patient was without some improvement. A total of eighty-three percent had excellent or good results. The niacin treatment was most effective in the more seriously ill chronic alcoholics. Niacinamide, another form of the vitamin, had no effect. This may be because niacin is a smaller molecule, more easily absorbed into the brain. Niacin also almost completely eliminated the "dry drunk syndrome", the hyperexcitable, manic episodes and serious potentially suicidal depressions experienced by many alcoholics on the wagon.

The dry drunk syndrome was first described in AA literature in 1962 and attributed to psychological factors. Hoffer and Osmond had noted that niacin treatment alleviated many of its distressing symptoms, such as irritability, aggressiveness, insomnia, fatigue, and nervousness. They attributed it to hypoglycemia, low blood sugar, which is found in most alcoholics. Alexander Schauss, in his book <u>Diet, Crime and Delinquency</u>, reported a 1973 study of two hundred alcoholics aged thirteen to eighty-two, in which ninety-seven percent were diagnosed hypoglycemic by a five or six-hour glucose tolerance test. Only eighteen percent of the controls in this study were hypoglycemic.

Recovering alcoholics frequently continue to overload their bodies with other toxic substances such as tobacco, caffeine, and large amounts of sugar. Meals are too often high in refined carbohydrates, fat and salt, and low in protein, fruits and vegetables, and whole grains. This type of diet produces and maintains the low blood sugar condition. The attempt to stave off alcohol craving by drinking coffee loaded with sugar, smoking tobacco, and keeping candy bars stashed for a quick lift, only aggravates the situation.

Both nicotine and caffeine stimulate adrenalin release, which raises blood sugar levels and gives a temporary lift. The body responds by producing excessive insulin, which pushes blood sugar down lower than it was before. When blood sugar drops, the brain is deprived of fuel and cannot

218

function normally. The person becomes confused and emotionally
unstable. He sweats, trembles, feels faint, and becomes depressed and
anxious. He feels a need to drink to supply quick energy. Since alcohol is
absorbed directly into the bloodstream without having to be digested,
alcoholics have learned that it gives the quickest relief. Although
hypoglycemia due to poor diet is one of the factors that can produce
alcoholism, excessive alcohol in turn can cause or aggravate
hypoglycemia. The damaged fatty liver is unable to store much glycogen
to be converted into glucose, and also has impaired ability to convert fat
and protein into glucose.

Changing to a wholesome, high protein diet free of sugar and white flour,
with supplemental B vitamins and minerals like zinc, manganese and
chromium, stabilizes blood sugar and mood swings, and attenuates the
desire for excessive caffeine and nicotine as well as alcohol. Adoption of
these principles could fit easily into the framework of AA and make their
work much easier.

Dr. David Hawkins of the North Nassau Mental Health Clinic in Long
Island, New York, has treated over six hundred alcoholics (as of 1982)
with a good diet and nutritional supplements. He used niacin and vitamin
C, 4000 mg or more of each per day, B6 50 mg, and vitamin E, 800 units
per day. The majority, seventy-one percent, showed marked
improvement. Most patients were able to recover and function in the
community with little or no professional help. Dr. Hawkins encountered
three recurrent problems among his patients that tended to complicate
recovery. One was the use of drugs such as sleeping pills, barbiturates
and tranquilizers. Another was hypoglycemia. On a six- hour glucose
tolerance test, many patients reported familiar feelings which they had had
in the past and which usually preceded a bout of drinking. Many patients
who had been sober for a long time still had periodic depression, tension,
anxiety, and desire to drink. These symptoms were eliminated by
correcting the low blood sugar.

The third problem which Dr. Hawkins found to complicate recovery was the presence of perceptual distortions -- misinterpretations of sensory perceptions of taste, smell, hearing, seeing, perception of body parts, and of space and time. These disperceptions were detected by a psychological test, the Hoffer-Osmond diagnostic test, or HOD, first developed by Hoffer and Osmond as a screening test for schizophrenia. A revised version of this test, called the Experimental World Inventory (EWI), is now more commonly used. These perceptual distortions are alleviated by treatment with niacin, B6, and other vitamins.

Another doctor who has successfully treated a great many alcoholics with nutrition is Nathan Brody. Dr. Brody specialized in the treatment of alcoholics for twenty-three years, at the Lakes Region General Hospital in New Hampshire. He tried everything, but had little success until he began using a nutritional approach. Then, he said, "Even the so-called failures respond and do better than the therapeutic successes of the past." He treated more than five hundred cases a year, and was chairman of the State Advisory Council on Alcoholism. Dr. Brody's treatment was based on biochemical analysis, and treatment with the specific nutrients required for each individual. It was essentially the same treatment that we used at the Princeton Brain Bio Center, based on blood tests for histamine level, vitamins and trace minerals.

Dr. Brody treated many alcoholics as outpatients, but severe cases had to be admitted to the hospital to begin treatment with detoxification. After drawing blood for sugar, alcohol level, histamine, and vitamin and mineral levels, patients were started on intravenous vitamin B complex and additional B6. In very sick patients the amounts were doubled. Intravenous vitamins were continued for at least five days, and vitamins by mouth were also given three times a day. When lab tests were completed, additional vitamins such as B12 and folic acid were added if necessary. Since seventy percent of Dr. Brody's patients experienced hypoglycemic symptoms, all patients were given a five-hour glucose tolerance test and put on a hypoglycemic diet.

In most cases, significant improvement was achieved within twenty-four hours. Librium or Thorazine was briefly prescribed, if necessary, for withdrawal symptoms. Patients were strongly encouraged to join AA, and AA meetings were held in the hospital. After discharge, patients were maintained on vitamins and good diet. Outpatients received the same treatment, without the IV vitamins. Dr Brody died in 1977, after successfully treating thousands of alcoholics. His effective nutritional treatment drew alcoholics from all over the northeast.

The significance of blood histamine level and trace mineral imbalances in treatment of schizophrenics was discovered by Dr. Carl Pfeiffer, while he directed the Bureau of Research in Neurology and Psychiatry at the New Jersey Neuropsychiatric Institute in Skillman, NJ. When the Bureau of Research was closed for lack of funds in 1972, Dr. Pfeiffer established the Brain Bio Center to continue his research on the biochemistry of schizophrenia and the development of nutritional treatments to correct the biochemical abnormalities. The same principles were applicable to treatment of alcoholism and many other disorders, and were used at the Bio Center to treat all types of mental illness, alcoholism, stress disorders, hyperactivity (ADD), etc. Since the Brain Bio Center was an outpatient clinic with no facilities for detoxification, we accepted only patients who were not currently drinking. We required all alcoholic patients to be active members of AA.

Patients accepted for treatment at the Brain Bio Center were given a battery of biochemical tests for blood histamine level, B12 and folic acid levels, blood tests for liver and kidney function, cholesterol, blood sugar, electrolytes, trace minerals, including copper, zinc, iron, manganese, and magnesium, urinalysis for sugar, protein and kryptopyrrole, and hair analysis for essential and toxic minerals. A complete medical history was taken, and a self-administered psychological test, the EWI (Experiential World Inventory), was given to detect disturbances in thought processes, perception, and mood.

The urinalysis included a test for kryptopyrolle or KP (previously called mauve factor or malvaria). An amount greater than 20 mcg% indicates a tendency to lose zinc and vitamin B6 in the urine, causing symptoms such as nervous exhaustion, emotional instability, nausea, and perceptual distortions, aggravated by stress. This condition, known as Pyroluria, responds quickly to zinc and B6 supplementation. Usually 30 mg of zinc twice a day was given, along with "enough B6 to produce normal dream recall."

Trace mineral levels were determined in all patients on both blood and hair samples. Almost all alcoholics were found to be deficient in zinc, and those with cirrhosis had the lowest levels. It is probable that zinc deficiency plays a role in the development of cirrhosis. Copper levels were often very high, especially when zinc was deficient. Copper is excitatory and in excess produces overstimulation of the brain, sometimes causing psychotic symptoms or severe depression. High copper is associated with liver damage and cirrhosis. Common sources of excess copper are copper plumbing, from which copper leaches into water standing in the pipes overnight, and commercial multivitamins with minerals. Zinc and copper are antagonistic, so zinc supplements will gradually bring down the copper level.

Copper forms part of the enzyme that destroys histamine, one of the neurotransmitters responsible for communication between brain cells. Excess copper produces a low histamine condition which Dr. Pfeiffer named Histapenia. This biochemical abnormality was found in about fifty percent of the schizophrenic patients treated at the Brain Bio Center. These patients had the common paranoid type of schizophrenia, with hallucinations, delusions, racing thoughts, paranoia and insomnia.

Alcoholics with low histamine are often subject to cyclic periods of depression and anxiety. They tend to be periodic drinkers who get intoxicated on weekends, as the tension of a job becomes unbearable by Friday night, or they indulge in a once a month binge. All patients at the Bio Center were tested for blood histamine level. Forty to seventy ng/ml was considered the normal range. Alcoholics and schizophrenics with low histamine and high copper were found to respond to treatment with niacin, B12 and folic acid. Niacin was given in amounts from 200 mg to 3 grams or more daily. At least 1 mg and up to 10 mg of folic acid was required. B12 was usually given by injection of 1 mg weekly. These patients also required zinc and manganese to lower the copper level and help build up histamine in the brain.

Dr. Pfeiffer's research found that people with the opposite problem, an excess of histamine (Histadelia), were the most prone to alcoholism. Histadelics have a high energy level, and tend to be Type A personalities, hard-driving, compulsive workaholics, with a tendency to depression, sometimes suicidal, and phobias. They have a high tolerance for alcohol and other drugs, and often find that prescription medications don't work unless prescribed in higher than normal amounts. They metabolize drugs and food rapidly and are sometimes compulsive eaters, but they usually accumulate little body fat, due to their fast metabolism.

A preliminary study of characteristics of high and low histamine people was done by Dr. Oscar Kruesi of Morristown, New Jersey. Ninety-one low histamine and ninety-seven high histamine people were surveyed. Fourteen percent of low histamine and twenty-eight percent of high histamine people reported having at least one drink a day. Only two percent of low histamine, but ten percent of high histamine people were alcoholic. According to Dr.Kruesi's survey, high histamine people required less sleep, had a higher sex drive, and were at least twice as high as low histamine people in incidence of allergies, asthma, duodenal ulcers, hypertension, and tension headaches, and seven times as high in incidence of migraine.

When high histamine people become alcoholic, they are usually hard-core, steady drinkers who seem to hold their liquor well and put away large amounts every day. Histadelia, like allergies, runs in families and may be associated not only with alcohol, but also abuse of other drugs. These people may be self-medicating with alcohol and drugs in an attempt to relieve their chronic depression. Some people subject to depression may have a lower than normal level of endorphin, a natural pain and anxiety-relieving brain chemical similar in structure to morphine. Such people would be easily addicted since drugs or alcohol make them feel more normal.

Dr. Pfeiffer speculated that the brilliant American playwright Eugene O'Neill may have been Histadelic. His illness was apparently hereditary. His immediate family tree, from both his paternal and maternal grandparents to his two sons, suffered from drug or alcohol addiction, severe depression, and in two cases, suicide. His mother was a morphine addict for twenty-five years, beginning at Eugene's birth, when it was prescribed for a very difficult delivery. One of O'Neill's sons became alcoholic and committed suicide. The other was a narcotic addict.

O'Neill harbored a compulsive personality, guilt feelings, and phobias of thunderstorms and crowds. He was preoccupied with a constant fear of insanity, endured deep and prolonged periods of depression, and had a volcanic inner tension. His suicidal tendencies were manifested by his self-destructive hard-core drinking and a single suicide attempt. A biographer described his long, narrow fingers, a physical characteristic of histadelics. (Dr. Pfeiffer believed this was an adaptation to dissipate the excess heat of fast oxidation.) At the age of thirty-seven, after his brother Jamie died of alcoholism, Eugene suddenly stopped drinking after a brief course of psychotherapy. But the depression (as portrayed in his tragedies) persisted until his death.

Histadelia can be diagnosed by a high blood histamine level or a high basophil count, and a careful metabolic history. Dr. Pfeiffer discovered how to lower histamine with calcium and the amino acid methionine in amounts of 500 mg of each twice a day. In difficult cases, the antiepileptic medication phenytoin (Dilantin) was used to bring the histamine down. Folic acid raises histamine so excessive amounts need to be avoided. Zinc and manganese are often needed also.

Another metabolic disorder that can be associated with alcoholism is cerebral allergy, an allergy to certain foods that affects the brain rather than causing the usual sneezing, wheezing, or rashes. One interesting case was a twenty-seven-year-old unmarried female school teacher who came to us with a history of several hospitalizations for alcoholism. She had joined AA after her second hospitalization, but a few months later she was still fighting hard to avoid her favorite alcoholic drinks.   Her histamine and copper were normal. She was not hypoglycemic. She was slightly pyroluric, which was corrected with 250 mg of B6 per day and a zinc supplement morning and night.

She was not aware of having any allergies, but craving a certain food or having a favorite food that is eaten very frequently, (in her case alcohol), is often an indication of an allergy to that food. Skin testing for allergies was done and she was found to be allergic to wheat, yeast, malt and rye, all common ingredients of alcoholic beverages. She did well on a twice weekly neutralizing injection for these foods, and the craving for alcohol soon diminished to a tolerable level.

Recommended Reading

Chapter 1 The Truth about Fat and Carbs

Atkins, Robert and Herwood, R W. <u>Dr Atkins' Diet Revolution</u>. New York: Bantam, 1972.
D'Adamo, Peter J, <u>Eat Right 4 Your Type</u>. New York: G P Putnam's Sons, 1996
Erasmo, Udo. <u>Fats that Heal Fats that Kill</u>.   Burnaby, BC, Canada: HarperCollins, 1999.
Ornish, Dean. <u>Dr. Dean Ornish's Program for Reversing Heart Disease.</u> New York: Ballentine, 1990
Pritikin, Nathan and McGrady, P. <u>The Pritikin Program for Diet and Exercise</u>. New York: Grosset and Dunlap, 1979

Chapter 2 Toxic Fat

Hyman, Mark. "Toxic Fat" <u>Alternative Therapies</u>. March/April 2007.
Robbins, John. <u>Diet for a New America</u>. Walpole, NH: Stillpoint, 1987
Steinman, David. <u>Diet for a Poisoned Planet</u>. New York: Harmony Books, 1990.

Chapter 3 Anti-Aging Food Rainbow

Carper, Jean. <u>The Food Pharmacy</u> Bantam Books, 1988.

Chapter 4 ThePescivore's Dilemma

Grescoe, Taras. <u>Bottom Feeders</u>. New York: Bloomsbury, 2008

Chapter 5 The China Study

Campbell, T. Colin. <u>The China Study</u>. Dallas, TX: Benbella, 2006

Chapter 6 Eating for A's

Schauss, Alexander, Meyer, Barbara F, and Meyer, Arnold. Eating for A's. New York: Pocket Books, 1991
Smith, Lendon. Feed Your Kids Right. New York: Dell, 1979

Chapter 7 Suppers for Sobriety

Larson, Joan M. Seven Weeks to Sobriety. New York: Ballantine Wellspring, 1997.
Ross, Julia. The Mood Cure. New York: Penguin, 2002.

Chapter 8 The Real Mediterranean Diet

Chapter 9 Chocolate

Waterhouse, Debra. Why Women Need Chocolate. New York: Hyperion, 1995

Chapter 10 Food and Mood

Schachter, Michael B. What Your Doctor May Not Tell You About Depression. New York: Warner Wellness, 2006.
Schwartz, George. Food Power. New York: McGraw-Hill, 1979.

Chapter 11 Brain Health and Longevity

Carper, Jean. Your Miracle Brain. New York: HarperCollins, 2000.
Crawford, Michael and Marsh, David. Nutrition and Evolution. New Haven, CT: Keats, 1995
Katz, Lawrence, and Rubin, Manning. Keep Your Brain Alive. New York: Workman, 1999.

Morgan, Elaine. <u>The Aquatic Ape</u>. New York: Stein and Day, 1982.
Schmukler, Alan. <u>Homeopathy, the Home Handbook for Survival</u>. 2003.
Singh Khalsa, Dharma. <u>Brain Longevity.</u> New York: Warner Books, 1999.

Chapter 12   Natural Treatment for Depression and Bipolar Disorder

Barnes, Broda and Galton, Lawrence. <u>Hypothyroidism, the Unsuspected Illness</u>. New York: Thomas Y. Crowell Company, 1976.
DeSchepper, Luc. <u>Human Condition: Critical</u>. Santa Fe, NM: Full of Life Publishing, 1993.
Guyol, Gracelyn. <u>Healing Depression and Bipolar Disorder without Drugs</u>. New York: Walker and Company, 2006.
Rudin, Donald and Felix, Clara. <u>The Omega-3 Phenomenon</u>. New York: Rawson Associates, 1987.
Slagle, Priscilla. <u>The Way Up From Down.</u> New York: St Martin's Press, 1987.
Stoll, Andrew, <u>The Omega-3 Connection</u>. New York: Simon and Schuster, 2001.

Chapter 13 Orthomolecular Psychiatry for Schizophrenia

Breggin, Peter. <u>Toxic Psychiatry</u>. New York: St. Martin's Press, 1991.
Edelman, Eva. <u>Natural Healing for Schizophrenia and Other Common Mental Disorders.</u> Eugene OR: Borage Books, 1998.
Hawkins, David and Pauling, Linus, editors, <u>Orthomolecular Psychiatry</u>. San Francisco: W. H. Freeman, 1973.
Hoffer, Abram and Osmond, Humphrey. <u>How to Live with Schizophrenia</u>. Secaucus, NJ: University Books, 1974.
Pauling, Linus. "Orthomolecular Psychiatry", <u>Science</u>. 19 April 1968, Volume 160, pp. 265-271
Pfeiffer, Carl C. <u>Mental and Elemental Nutrients</u>. New Canaan, CT: Keats Publishing, 1975.
Pfeiffer, Carl C. <u>Zinc and Other Micronutrients</u>. New Canaan, CT: Keats Publishing, 1978.

Pfeiffer, Carl C. Nutrition and Mental Illness. Rochester, VT: Healing Arts Press, 1987.
Pfeiffer, Carl C. The Schizophrenas, Ours to Conquer. Wichita KS: Bio-Commmunications Press, 1988.
Wells, Brian. Psychedelic Drugs. New York: Jason Aronson, 1974

Chapter 14 Autism and Mercury

Bettleheim, Bruno. The Empty Fortress. New York: Free Press, 1967.
Lansky, Amy. Impossible Cure: The Promise of Homeopathy. Portola Valley, CA: R L Ranch Press, 2003.
Pangborn, Jon and Baker, Sidney. Autism: Effective Biomedical Treatments. Boston: DAN!, 2005.
Olmsted, Dan and Blaxill, Mark. The Age of Autism. New York: Thomas Dunne Books, St. Martin's Press, 2010

Handley, J B.How to End the Autism Epidemic. Chelsea, Vermont: Chelsea Green Pub Co, 2018

Chapter 15 Heavy Metal Brain Damage

Brownstein, David. Iodine. West Bloonfield, MI: Medical Arts Press, 2008.
Levitt, Steven and Dubner, Stephen. Freakonomics. New York: HarperCollins, 2006.
Schauss, Alexander. Diet, Crime and Delinquency. Berkeley, CA: Parker House, 1980
Simontacchi, Carol. The Crazy Makers. New York: Jeremy P. Tarcher/Putnam, 2000.
Wenzel, Klaus-Georg and Pataraccia, Raymond. The Earth's Gift to Medicine. Alton, ON, Canada: KOS Publishing, Inc, 2005.

Chapter 16 Natural Help for Arthritis

Brown, Ellen. <u>Healing Joint Pain Naturally</u>. New York: Broadway Books, 2001.
Hahnemann, Samuel. <u>Organon of Medicine, Sixth Edition</u>, translated by William Boericke. New Delhi: B. Jain Publishers, Ltd, 1990.

Chapter 17 Prevent Breast Cancer with Ayurveda

Horner, Christine. <u>Waking the Warrior Goddess</u>. Laguna Beach, CA: Basic Health Publications, 2007.
Weed, Susun. <u>Breast Cancer? Breast Health!</u>. Woodstock, NY: Ash Tree Publishing, 1996.

Chapter 18 Flu Alternatives

Balch, Phyllis and Balch,James. <u>Prescription for Nutritional Healing, Third Edition</u>. New York: Avery, 2000.
Barry, John. <u>The Great Influenza</u>. London: Penguin Books Ltd, 2005.
Shepherd, Dorothy. <u>Homoeopathy in Epidemic Diseases</u>. Essex, England: C.W. Daniel Company Ltd, 1967.

Chapter 19   What is Homeopathy?

Coulter, Harris. <u>Homeopathic Science and Modern Medicine</u> Berkeley, CA: North Atlantic Books, 1980.
Ullman, Dana. <u>The Consumer's Guide to Homeopathy</u>. New York: Tarcher/Putnam, 1995.
Vithoulkas, George. <u>Homeopathy Medicine for the New Millennium</u>. New York: The International Academy of Classical Homeopathy, 2000.

Chapter 20   Homeopathy for Children's Illnesses

Herscu, Paul. The Homeopathic Treatment of Children. Berkeley, CA: North Atlantic Books, 1991.
Ullman, Dana. Homeopathy for Children and Infants. New York: J.P. Tarcher/Perigee, 1992.

Chapter 21 Homeopathy for Attention and Behavior Problems

Reichenberg-Ullman, Judyth and Ullman, Robert, Ritalin-Free Kids. Rocklin, CA: Prima Publishing, 1996.

Chapter 22   Homeopathy for Depression

De Schepper, Luc. Human Condition: Critical. Santa Fe, NM: Full of Life Publishing, 1993.
Smith, Trevor, Homoeopathy for Psychological Illness. Sussex, England: Worthing

Chapter 23 Homeopathy for Anxiety, Fear, and Phobias

Chappell, Peter. Emotional Healing with Homeopathy. Rockport, MA: Element, Inc., 1994.
Nauman, Eileen. Poisons that Heal. Sedona, AZ: Light Technology Publishing, 1995.

Chapter 24 Homeopathy for Anger, Irritability and Rage

Castro, Miranda. Homeopathic Guide to Stress. New York: St. Martin's Griffin, 1996.

Chapter 25 Homeopathy for Women's Problems

Colborn, Theo, Dumanoski, Dianne and Myers, John. Our Stolen Future. New York: Plume, 1997.

Handley, Rima. Homoeopathy for Women. London: Thorsons, 1993.
Lee, John R and Hopkins, Virginia. What your Doctor May Not Tell You About Menopause. New York: Warner, 1996.
Somers, Suzanne. The Sexy Years. New York: Crown, 2004.
Speight, Phyllis. Homoeopathic Remedies for Women's Ailments. Essex, England: C.W. Daniel Company Ltd, 1985.

Chapter 26   Homeopathy for First Aid and Natural Disasters

Kruzel, Thomas, The Homeopathic Emergency Guide. Berkeley, CA: North Atlantic Books, 1992.
Shepherd, Dorothy. Homeopathy for the First Aider. Essex, England: C.W. Daniel Company Ltd, 1953.

Chapter 27 Light and Health

Douglass, William, Into the Light. Dunwoody, GA: Second Opinion Press, 1993.
Gross, Michael. Light and Life. New York: Oxford University Press, 2002.
Liberman, Jacob. Light – Medicine of the Future. Santa Fe, NM: Bear and Company, 1991.

Chapter 28 Weather, Cycles and Health, Our Cosmic Connection

Thomas, Pat. Under the Weather. London: Fusion Press, 2004.

Chapter 29   Climate Truth

Gore, Al. An Inconvenient Truth. (movie) Hollywood, CA: Paramount, 2006.

Chapter 30 No Nukes Now

Caldicott, Helen. Nuclear Power is Not the Answer. New York: New Press, 2006.

Chapter 31 Seafood and Evolution

Morgan, Elaine. <u>The Aquatic Ape</u>. New York: Stein and Day, 1982.
Morgan, Elaine. <u>The Descent of Woman</u>. New York: Bantam Books, 1972.

Chapter 32 Blood Type and Evolution

D'Adamo, Peter. <u>Live Right for Your Type</u>. New York: G.P. Putnam's Sons, 2001.
Sjoo, Monica and Mor, Barbara. <u>The Great Cosmic Mother</u>. San Francisco: Harper and Row, 1987.

Chapter 33 Evolution – Two Paths

Bakan, Joel. <u>The Corporation</u>. New York: Free Press, 2004.
DeWaal, Frans, and Lanting, Frans. <u>Bonobo the Forgotten Ape</u>. Berkeley, CA: University of California Press, 1997.
Eisler, Rianne. <u>The Chalice and the Blade</u>. San Francisco: Harper and Row, 1987.
Sagan, Carl. <u>The Dragons of Eden</u>. New York: Ballantine Books, 1977.
Sagan, Carl. <u>The Varieties of Scientific Experience</u>. New York: Penguin Press, 2006.
Wrangham, Richard. <u>Demonic Males</u>. Boston: Houghton Mifflin, 1996.

Chapter 34 Helper's High and Winner's High

Darwin, Charles. <u>Descent of Man</u>. New York: A. L. Burt, 1874.
Darwin, Charles. <u>The Origin of Species</u>. New York: Mentor Books, 1958.
Dyer, Wayne. <u>The Power of Intention</u>. Carlsbad, CA: Hay House, 2004.
Gray, John. <u>Men are from Mars, Women are from Venus</u>. New York: HarperCollins, 1992.

Chapter 35 Art and Science , Heart and Silence of Breath

Fehmi, Les. <u>The Open Focus Brain</u>. Boston: Shambala, 2007.
Pearsall, Paul. <u>Wishing Well</u>. New York: Hyperion, 2000.
Pert, Candace. <u>Molecules of Emotion</u>. New York: Scribner, 1997.
Schlain, Leonard. <u>The Alphabet Versus the Goddess</u>. New York: Viking, 1998.
Silva, Jose. <u>You the Healer</u>. Tiburon, CA: H J Kramer Inc, 1989.

Afterword: Natural vs Synthetic, Herb vs Drug

Herer, Jack. <u>The Emperor Wears No Clothes</u>. Van Nuys, CA: HEMP Publishing, 1991.